MOCKTAILS OVER COCKTAILS

DISCOVER HOW TO MANAGE ALCOHOL CONSUMPTION, ENJOY BETTER HEALTH, IMPROVE MENTAL CLARITY, AND SAVE MONEY. SIMPLE STRATEGIES FOR A SUCCESSFUL DRY JANUARY AND SOBER OCTOBER.

BEYOND THE BAR PRESS

CONTENTS

1st Editon

Publisher: Beyond the Bar Press

INTRODUCTION

Once upon a time, in the not-so-distant past, there was a guy named Mike. Mike loved his Friday night drinks with friends. It was a ritual. Two beers turned into three, and sometimes into a blurry memory and a Saturday morning headache. It felt normal until one January when Mike decided to try this thing called "Dry January." The first week was tough. He missed the clinking glasses and the easy laughter. But as days turned into weeks, something magical happened. Mike felt sharper, as if he had upgraded his brain's software. He saved money, lost a few pounds, and realized he didn't need a drink to have a good time. By February, Mike was a new man; his story is just one of many.

The purpose of this book is simple. It's your guide to navigating Dry January, Sober October, and any other month you choose to go dry. Whether you're sober curious or just looking to hit the reset button, this book will help you manage your alcohol consumption, improve your health, gain mental clarity, and save some serious cash.

Allow me to introduce myself. I'm your friendly guide on this journey. I've spent over 20 years in the alcohol beverage industry, witnessing firsthand the impact alcohol can have on our lives. My passion lies in helping people like you overcome the challenges associated with drinking and discover a healthier, more fulfilling lifestyle.

Now, let's talk about why Dry January (or even Sober October) is worth your time. Studies show that taking a break from alcohol can lead to improved liver function, better sleep, and even weight loss. Financially, cutting out those drinks can save you hundreds of dollars a month. Did you know that the average person spends over $500 a year on alcohol? That's a nice vacation fund right there.

This book is for health-conscious, curious adults or those just ready for a change. Maybe you're seeking support or personal growth or want to see if you can do it. You're in the right place. We'll tackle your everyday concerns and give you the tools to succeed.

Here's a quick overview of what you'll find in this book. We'll start with tips for preparing for your dry month, including how to handle social situations without feeling like a party pooper. Then, we'll dive into delicious mocktail recipes—over 50—to keep your taste buds happy. We'll also cover financial savings strategies and personal growth tips to ensure you come out of this experience better than ever.

What makes this book unique? Well, it's not just about abstaining from alcohol. It's about embracing a new lifestyle for a month and seeing where it takes you. With practical advice, mocktail recipes, and strategies for personal growth, this book offers a fresh perspective on going dry.

This book teaches you how to manage your drinking habits, boost your health, sharpen your mind, and save money. You'll feel empowered to take control of your life and make positive changes.

I encourage you to engage with this book actively. Use it as a workbook. Reflect, journal, and apply the strategies we discuss. The more you put into it, the more you'll get out of it.

So, here's your call to action: Commit to a dry month. Pick up this book and let it be your trusted guide. Take the first step towards a healthier lifestyle and see what amazing things happen when you go dry.

SETTING THE STAGE FOR SUCCESS

Y ou know that moment when you first wake up, feeling like you've got a hundred-pound weight sitting on your head, and you swear to yourself, "Never again"? Well, let me introduce you to Sarah. She was the queen of the "just one more" crowd, always up for a good time but often regretting it the next day. Then came her first Dry January. She started it as a joke, a dare among friends. But as the days went by, she noticed something. Her skin glowed, her jeans fit better, and she could actually remember everything from the previous night's Netflix binge. Suddenly, Sarah was thriving. Her story is a reminder that taking a break from alcohol can lead to unexpected, yet delightful, surprises.

UNDERSTANDING THE SOBER CURIOUS MOVEMENT

The sober curious movement is like that cool, mysterious neighbor who moved in next door and suddenly everyone wants to be friends with. This trend was sparked in 2018 by Ruby Warrington's book, "Sober Curious," which invited people to explore sobriety without the pressure of giving up alcohol forever. It's all about asking, "What if I don't drink?" and seeing where that question leads. This movement has picked up steam thanks to social media platforms like Instagram and TikTok, with hashtags and communities popping up to support those choosing to sip on life instead of a glass of wine. People from all walks of life are joining in, sharing their stories, and normalizing the idea that it's okay to question our drinking habits.

Being sober curious doesn't mean you have to ditch the booze for good. It's more about curiosity than commitment. It's about exploring what sobriety feels like, without the pressure of a lifelong vow. Imagine walking into a party and having the freedom to choose whether to drink or not based on how you feel, not on social expectations. The appeal here is undeniable. With wellness trends booming, more people are tuning into their health and realizing the benefits of taking a break from alcohol. Not only does it promise clearer skin and better sleep, but it also offers a mental refresh. Socially, it allows you to be present, really savor those conversations, and who knows, you might even remember the punchline to that joke you've been trying to recall.

The real beauty of the sober curious movement is its inclusivity. It's a judgment-free zone where anyone can join, whether you're a weekend warrior looking to cut back or someone who wants to see how life feels on the other side of the cocktail glass. There are no rigid rules dictating how you should proceed. It's more of an open invitation to explore your relationship with alcohol on your terms, surrounded by a community that gets it.

Explore Your Curiosity

Take a moment to reflect: What does being sober curious mean to you? Is it about health, clarity, or perhaps a financial break? Grab a journal and jot down your thoughts. This isn't about setting rules; it's about understanding your motivations and what you hope to gain by reducing your alcohol intake. Reflect on what this means for you and how you envision incorporating this curiosity into your life.

THE HEALTH BENEFITS OF GOING ALCOHOL-FREE

Remember those mornings when you wake up feeling like your brain was replaced with a brick? That's the magic of alcohol, folks. But something pretty amazing happens when you decide to give your liver a break. Your liver, working overtime to process all those cocktails, can finally kick back and take a breather. This organ is like the body's detox powerhouse, and when it's not busy handling alcohol, it can focus on doing its real job: keeping you healthy. Say goodbye to that perpetual grogginess and hello to a body that functions like a well-oiled machine. It's like giving your liver a spa day every day.

And let's talk about sleep. That elusive, glorious thing we all crave yet often messes up with a few too many nightcaps. Alcohol might make you feel sleepy, but it messes with your sleep cycle, especially REM sleep, which is the kind of deep sleep that makes you wake up feeling like you're ready to conquer the world. When you cut out alcohol, your body finally gets the chance to rest properly, leading to better sleep quality. Imagine waking up refreshed, not needing three cups of coffee to feel human. Your mornings could be less about hitting snooze and more about feeling like you've just woken up from a fairy tale nap.

I know what you're thinking: "But what about my energy levels?" When you remove alcohol from the equation, you'll likely notice a surge in your energy. Suddenly, those mid-afternoon slumps might start to disappear. You might find yourself bouncing through the day, tackling to-do lists with the vigor of a kid in a candy store. With improved sleep and a liver that's not constantly in emergency mode, your body can channel its energy into things that actually matter, like living life to the fullest.

Mentally, the benefits are just as compelling. Alcohol can be a sneaky thief, robbing you of mental clarity and emotional stability. Removing it from your life can lead to a noticeable reduction in anxiety and depression symptoms. Your brain gets a break from the rollercoaster of highs and lows, settling into a more stable, happy place. Your cognitive functions sharpen up, like turning up the resolution of a blurry picture.

Conversations become more engaging, decisions clearer, and who knows, you might even start winning at trivia night.

Weight management is another delightful perk. Alcohol is packed with empty calories that can quickly add up, leading to those pesky extra pounds. By cutting out alcohol, you're not only reducing your calorie intake but also making room for healthier food choices. Your body starts processing nutrients better, and that pizza slice you had last night might actually give you energy instead of regret. The scale might start moving in the right direction, and those jeans that used to pinch are suddenly a little more forgiving.

Let's not forget the overall boost to well-being. Your immune system, which was probably getting a bit sluggish, gets a chance to beef up. Without alcohol weighing it down, your body can fend off colds and other nasties with gusto. Your skin also joins the party, clearing up and glowing like you've just returned from a fancy spa retreat. You'll notice fewer breakouts, more hydration, and a complexion that screams vitality. It's like your entire body gets a software update, and you're suddenly running on the latest version of you.

Reflect on Your Health Goals

Take a moment to jot down your own health goals. How do you envision your life-changing without alcohol? What are the physical and mental benefits you're most excited about? Grab a notepad and consider writing a health wish list. This isn't just about what you're giving up but what you're gaining—a healthier, happier you.

FINANCIAL GAINS OF QUITTING ALCOHOL

Who doesn't love the idea of a little extra cash in their pocket? When you quit drinking, the financial benefits can be nothing short of spectacular. Imagine this: the average person can spend anywhere from $260 to $780 a year if they're having just one to three drinks a week. Now, bump that up to a daily habit, and you might be looking at over $3,000 a year. That's like a small fortune, enough to fund a dream vacation or upgrade that outdated couch you've been eyeing. The savings don't stop at the bar tab, either. Cutting back on alcohol means fewer spontaneous nights out and lower tabs at restaurants, which often mark up drink prices to an absurd degree. It's like finding a hole in your wallet and finally stitching it up.

Beyond the direct savings are the sneaky, indirect financial perks of saying goodbye to booze. First, let's talk about healthcare. Alcohol doesn't just cost you at the bar; it can sneak into your doctor's office bills, too. By drinking less, you might find fewer visits to the doc for those pesky ailments that seem to pop up after a night out. Your health insurance premiums might not drop immediately, but a healthier life-style can reduce medical expenses over time. Then there's the fact you won't be needing those late-night rideshares after a few too many. Not only does this save money, but it also spares you the hassle of the dreaded "Where did I park?" game.

So, what do you do with all this extra dough? The possibilities are endless, but here's a thought: reallocate your newfound savings towards something fulfilling. Have you always wanted to take up photography? Now you can afford that fancy camera. Are you eyeing a pottery class? Go for it. The money you save can be an investment in hobbies or personal growth, things that enrich your life far beyond the temporary buzz of a drink. You might even set aside a little for that special treat—a weekend getaway or a spa day, perhaps. It's about rewarding yourself meaningfully and contributing to your happiness and well-being.

Let's not forget the broader impact on your financial health. Those savings can be the boost you need to build an emergency fund, providing a safety net for unexpected expenses. Or maybe it's time to tackle those pesky debts lingering in the background. Paying off credit cards or student loans relieves stress and frees up your future income for things that truly matter to you. The financial freedom from reducing alcohol consumption isn't just about cutting costs; it's about gaining control over your financial destiny.

SETTING REALISTIC AND ACHIEVABLE GOALS

Let's say you're standing on the edge of a pool, toes curling over the edge, ready to dive in. But wait! Before you leap, you need a plan, right? That's where goal setting comes into play. It's like plotting your course on a treasure map, ensuring you hit all the right spots without wandering. Enter the SMART goals framework - Specific, Measurable, Achievable, Relevant, and Time-bound. It's a way to ensure your goals aren't just dreams but realistic targets you can hit. For instance, instead of saying, "I'll drink less," make it specific: "I'll limit myself to two drinks a week." Measure it by tracking your intake. Ensure it's achievable by setting a limit that feels doable. Keep it relevant to your broader life goals, like improving health or saving money. And set a time frame—say, a month—to keep yourself on track.

Breaking down these goals into smaller steps is critical. Imagine you're building a Lego castle. You wouldn't try to assemble the whole thing at once, would you? No, you'd start with the foundation and work your way up. The same goes for your goals. Let's say your big goal is to cut down on alcohol. Start with manageable steps like skipping the Monday night drink or replacing your weekend cocktail with a mocktail. It's about making progress, brick by brick until you've built something solid and impressive.

Success isn't a one-size-fits-all concept. It's deeply personal, like your favorite pizza topping. For some, success might mean going a whole month without a drop. For others, it might be simply cutting back to weekends. Define what success looks like for you and set short-term milestones to keep you motivated. Celebrate those small wins—maybe with a non-alcoholic treat or a relaxing evening doing something you love. Recognizing these victories fuels your motivation and makes the journey enjoyable.

Tracking progress is where the rubber meets the road. There needs to be more than just setting goals; you must know how you're doing. Use apps or good old-fashioned journals to log your progress. There's something satisfying about seeing your achievements laid out in black and white. You may opt for a weekly check-in with a friend or accountability partner. They can offer encouragement or a gentle nudge if you start to stray. It's like having a personal cheerleader, minus the pom-poms.

Flexibility plays a crucial role in goal setting. Life isn't static, and neither should your goals be. If you find yourself struggling, it's okay to reassess and realign your objectives. Maybe you aimed to cut down to one drink a week but found it too challenging. Adjust it to two drinks and see how that feels. The key is to be kind to yourself during setbacks. Remember, it's not about perfection but progress. You can adjust your plan as you learn what works best for you.

THE SCIENCE BEHIND ALCOHOL AND YOUR BODY

Alcohol is like that uninvited party guest who overstays their welcome. It might initially seem harmless, but the story changes once it starts making rounds in your body. The liver, your body's detox superstar, takes the brunt of the work. It's tasked with breaking down alcohol into non-toxic compounds, a job that keeps it busy for hours. Over time, excessive drinking can lead to fatty liver, inflammation, and even cirrhosis. Then there's the brain, which faces neurotransmitter disruptions, leading to that familiar foggy feeling. In the short term, alcohol can impair judgment and coordination. Long-term, it might contribute to memory problems and mental health issues. Your heart, stomach, and pancreas aren't spared either, as they face increased risks of high blood pressure, ulcers, and pancreatitis. It's a cascade of effects that can leave your body feeling like it's been through a marathon, even if you've only been binge-watching your favorite series.

Giving your body a break from alcohol is like sending it on a much-needed holiday. Detoxification is the body's way of hitting the reset button. Initially, you might face withdrawal symptoms like headaches or irritability as your body adjusts. But hang tight because things will improve. Your liver gets a chance to heal, and your brain chemistry balances out. Over time, you might notice increased energy levels, better digestion, and a clearer mind. It's a reminder of the human body's resilience when given a chance to recuperate. This break from alcohol is not just about abstaining; it's about allowing your body to thrive without the constant battle against toxins.

But let's not sugarcoat it—excessive drinking comes with a host of adverse effects. Experts consistently highlight the dangers of excessive drinking. According to numerous studies, individuals who drink heavily face a higher risk of mortality and health complications. The Centers for Disease Control and Prevention (CDC) states that excessive alcohol use can lead to chronic diseases, including high blood pressure, heart disease, stroke, liver disease, and digestive problems. It's like signing up for a club you definitely don't want to be a part of. Mentally, alcohol can act as a depressant, exacerbating anxiety and depression. It can cloud your thinking and impair decision-making, turning even the simplest tasks into Herculean efforts. Over time, this can impact your mental health and overall cognitive function. Dr. Harrison, a leading researcher in alcohol-related health issues, explains, "Alcohol can be a silent saboteur, affecting nearly every organ in the body. It's crucial to understand the risks and make informed choices."

The statistics are sobering, to say the least, but they underscore the importance of understanding what alcohol does to our bodies. Taking a break from it isn't just a test of willpower; it's a step towards a healthier, more balanced life.

2

UNDERSTANDING DRY JANUARY

O nce upon a time, in a bustling office in the UK, Emily decided she needed a break from the usual holiday indulgence. She had a half marathon looming, and those late-night glasses of wine were starting to feel like lead in her sneakers. So, she made a bold choice: to go alcohol-free for the entire month of January. Little did Emily know that her personal challenge would spark a movement now known globally as Dry January. Fast forward to today, and what started as a personal resolution has grown into a phenomenon with thousands participating annually, all inspired by Emily's quest for clarity and fitness.

WHAT IS DRY JANUARY?

Dry January, officially launched by Alcohol Change UK in 2013, is a commitment to abstain from alcohol for January. It's like hitting the reset button on your relationship with booze, giving your liver a chance to thank you profusely. The goals are simple but profound: to reassess the role of alcohol in your life, explore the benefits of temporary abstinence, and engage in some solid self-reflection. The idea is to see how life feels without the evening glass of wine and learn about yourself in the process. It's like taking your liver on a vacation it didn't know it needed.

Participation in Dry January has skyrocketed over the years, with a community that spans the globe. From its humble beginnings with 4,000 participants, it now boasts a crowd of over 175,000 and counting. The appeal is in its simplicity, and the community support it offers. There's a certain camaraderie in knowing you're part of a worldwide effort, all striving for better health and clearer minds, if only for a month. And let's not forget those shared struggles and triumphant cheers when you make it through that first Friday night pub crawl sans pint.

While Dry January stands tall as the poster child for alcohol-free months, it's not alone. Sober October is another popular choice, offering a similar challenge but in the crisp autumn air. The main difference? Timing. While January is about shaking off the holiday excess, October is a chance to embrace a healthier lifestyle as the year winds down. Both offer unique aspects and community support, so whether you're a January warrior or an October abstainer, there's a place for you.

The Dry January experience is a journey with a unique rhythm. The first week might feel like climbing a steep hill, where your usual routines challenge your resolve. By the second week, you'll likely find your groove, with motivation building, as you notice subtle changes— better sleep, clearer thoughts, maybe even a spring in your step. Expect a sense of accomplishment and perhaps a new perspective on your habits by month's end. It's a chance to reflect on what you've learned and decide what, if anything, you'd like to carry forward.

Reflect on Your Dry January Goals

As you enter Dry January, take some time to jot down what you hope to achieve. Are you looking to reset your habits, save some cash, or just see if you can do it? Write it down and revisit it throughout the month. This isn't just a challenge; it's a chance to learn about yourself.

PREPARING MENTALLY FOR DRY JANUARY

Imagine your mind as a garden filled with growth potential. You need to cultivate the right mindset to make the most of Dry January. Picture this month not as a deprivation but an opportunity to plant seeds of change. Instead of focusing on what you're giving up, think about what you're gaining: clearer nights, fresher mornings, and the chance to explore life without a drink in hand. Setting a positive tone from the start can make all the difference. Try using affirmations, those little pep talks you whisper to yourself. "I am choosing health and happiness" or "I am open to change" can work wonders. These affirmations are mental anchors, keeping you steady when the waters get choppy.

Now, let's talk preparation. Visualization exercises are like mental dress rehearsals. Close your eyes and see yourself thriving through Dry January. Imagine each day, each moment, as if it happened successfully. Feel the clarity, the energy, the sense of achievement. Visualization isn't just woo-woo talk; it's a technique athletes use to prepare for the big game. Pair this with some good old-fashioned journaling, where you can pen down your intentions and goals for the month. Capture your hopes, your challenges, and your strategies. It's like having a roadmap guiding you through the maze of temptations and triumphs.

Finding your motivation is like uncovering your personal treasure map. What's your "X marks the spot"? For some, it might be health goals, like waking up without the foggy remnants of the night before. Others might be driven by the financial aspect, looking to save a few bucks for that concert ticket or weekend getaway. Then there are those of us who see it as a chance for personal growth, to learn more about ourselves, and to push our boundaries. Whatever it is, knowing your motivation gives you a reason to push through when the allure of a cold beer on a Friday night seems a little too tempting.

Building a support plan is like assembling your team of cheerleaders minus the pom-poms. Whether it's friends joining the challenge or family members understanding your goals, having a support system can make all the difference. Let them know why you're doing this and how they can help. Maybe it's joining you for a mocktail night or skipping the usual pub crawl. Don't forget about the digital world, either. Online groups and forums can provide a wealth of support, from sharing tips to knowing others are in the same boat. This is your time, your month. Whether you're motivated by the promise of a healthier you or the allure of a fatter wallet, embracing a positive mindset can turn Dry January from a daunting challenge into a rewarding adventure.

SETTING YOUR INTENTIONS AND GOALS

Have you ever thought about why you're jumping into Dry January? I mean, really thought about it? Setting clear intentions is like laying down a roadmap before a road trip. It gives direction and meaning, turning what might feel like a daunting task into a purposeful endeavor. Personal motivations are your compass. Maybe you're here to shed a couple of pounds, or perhaps you've noticed your wallet feels lighter after weekends out. Some folks want to see if they can do it, like a personal Everest. Whatever your reason, knowing it can be the difference between giving up halfway and pushing through with gusto. Long-term benefits are where the magic happens. Setting intentions isn't just about getting through January; it's about creating lasting change. It's about waking up in February with a newfound appreciation for mornings or a few extra bucks in your pocket.

Achieving goals is an art; the SMART framework is your brush and canvas. Specific goals mean you're not just saying, "I want to drink less," but rather, "I'll only drink at social events." Measurable means you can track your progress, maybe by how many days you go without a drink. Achievable is key; setting a goal that's within reach ensures you're not setting yourself up for failure. Relevant ties back to your intentions. Why are you doing this? Finally, Time-bound gives you that deadline—January 31st, in this case. Short-term goals keep you motivated as you see quick wins, while long-term goals ensure you're building habits that last beyond January.

Self-reflection is your best friend in this process. Grab a journal and start scribbling. Ask yourself, "Why do I drink?" "What do I hope to gain from this month?" "How do I feel about my drinking habits?" These questions aren't meant to judge but to understand. They're like a flashlight in a dark room, helping you see things clearly. Writing down your thoughts is cathartic and revealing. It's a moment to pause and think, to understand yourself better, and to set the stage for change.

Your Turn: Set Your Own Goals

Take a moment to jot down your own goals for Dry January. Use the SMART framework to ensure they're clear and achievable. Reflect on what you hope to gain-better health, financial savings, or the satisfaction of doing something challenging. This isn't just about stopping a habit; it's about starting something new.

3

BUILDING A SUPPORT SYSTEM

Imagine you're an adventurer setting out on a quest. Would you go it alone, relying solely on your wits and a trusty map? Or would you gather a band of merry companions to cheer you on, share some laughs, and maybe carry the snacks? The answer should be obvious. A supportive community isn't just a nice-to-have; it's your secret weapon in this dry endeavor. Having a network of folks who understand what you're going through is like having a safety net when walking that tightrope of temptation. They keep you accountable, providing gentle nudges when your resolve wavers. And let's face it, there's immense comfort in knowing you're not the only one longing for a cold brew on a Friday night.

FINDING YOUR DRY TRIBE: ONLINE AND LOCAL SUPPORT GROUPS

Online support groups have become the modern-day campfire where people gather to share stories, advice, and the occasional virtual high-five. Platforms like Reddit's r/stopdrinking offer a space for individuals to connect, share their triumphs and challenges, and offer encouragement to one another. Then there's the Dry January® Community

Group on Facebook, a bustling hub of like-minded individuals all committed to making it through the month without a drop. It's a place to post about your progress, ask for advice, or vent about how your office keeps hosting happy hours. The camaraderie and encouragement found in these groups can be inspiring.

Locally, you might find support in places you wouldn't have thought to look. Community centers and wellness clubs often host meet-ups or events focused on healthy living, including alcohol-free lifestyles. These gatherings provide an opportunity to meet new people on a similar path, offering accountability and friendship. If you're seeking a more structured approach, consider checking out local Alcoholics Anonymous (AA) groups. While AA traditionally supports those seeking long-term sobriety, many chapters welcome those looking to take a temporary break. It's all about finding what works for you in your local scene.

Engaging with these communities can significantly enhance your experience. Start by sharing your story. Be open about your goals and challenges; you'll likely find others who relate. Attend virtual or in-person meet-ups to forge connections and gain support. It's like being part of a team where everyone is rooting for each other to cross the finish line. Remember, the more you put into these communities, the more you'll get out of them. So go ahead, dive in, and discover the strength from knowing you're not alone on this path.

To get the most out of your community experience, consider creating a list of online and local groups to explore. Jot down their names, meeting times, and any relevant contact information. Use this as a roadmap to guide your engagement, helping you stay connected and supported throughout your alcohol-free adventure.

HOW TO HAVE HONEST CONVERSATIONS WITH FRIENDS AND FAMILY

Picture this: you're gearing up to have "the talk" with your nearest and dearest, but instead of it being the dreaded birds and bees, it's about your decision to tackle Dry January. Timing is everything. Choose a moment when everyone is relaxed, maybe after a cozy dinner or leisurely walk. Avoid the hustle and bustle of a busy day or the chaos of a family gathering. A quiet, comfortable setting can make all the difference. Now, on to the words themselves. Be transparent and honest. You don't need to write a speech, but having a few key points in mind can help. "I've decided to take a break from alcohol for a month to see how it affects my health" is a simple, straightforward way to start. Follow it up with, "I'd appreciate your support as I try something new." This approach sets a positive tone and opens the door to dialogue.

Now, brace yourself for the reactions. Your loved ones might have a few questions or concerns. Some might fear this is a prelude to a permanent lifestyle overhaul and start imagining a world without your famous party dance moves. Reassure them by emphasizing the temporary nature of your challenge. Explain your motivations without coming across as judgmental about their choices. It's about you, after all, not them. "I'm doing this for my health and to see what changes I notice," you might say. This keeps the focus on your journey and avoids any unintended finger-pointing.

Maintaining those social ties without alcohol can be a bit of a balancing act, but it's absolutely doable. Suggest alternative activities that don't revolve around drinks. How about a hiking day, a cooking class, or even a good old-fashioned game night? Highlight the importance of spending time together, reminding them that you cherish their company, not the contents of your glass. "Let's catch up over brunch this weekend," you could propose. The goal is to keep the connection strong, even if the setting looks slightly different.

Conversation Starters

To help break the ice, consider using some conversation starters. "I've been thinking about trying Dry January. What do you think?" or "I heard about this thing called Dry January. Have you ever considered it?" can open up a discussion. These prompts encourage dialogue and can lead to a supportive conversation where your loved ones feel included in your decision.

CREATING A SUPPORTIVE HOME ENVIRONMENT

Imagine your home as your oasis during Dry January. It should be where you feel relaxed, encouraged, and ready to tackle this month with gusto. Start by giving your space a little makeover. Remove any alcohol and related paraphernalia that might tempt you during a moment of weakness. You know, those wine glasses that seem to wink at you every time you open the cupboard. Clearing them out, or at least tucking them away, helps create a booze-free zone. Next, stock up on non-alcoholic beverages. Fill your fridge with sparkling water, juices, and maybe some fancy kombucha. This way, when the craving hits, you've got a refreshing alternative at the ready.

Let's talk about getting your housemates or family involved. This isn't just your challenge; it can be a fun, collective effort. Set shared goals, like cooking a new recipe together each week or planning a weekend activity that doesn't involve alcohol. Maybe it's a hike, a trip to the museum, or even a DIY spa day at home. Brainstorm together to come up with a list of things everyone can enjoy. You build a support network under your roof by involving those you live with. Who doesn't love an excuse to try something new and exciting? It makes the experience feel less like a chore and more like an adventure.

Adding some visual and motivational aids around the house can be surprisingly effective. Think of it as decorating with purpose. Put up posters or write quotes that inspire you. "One day at a time" or "You got this!" can serve as daily reminders of your resolve. Progress charts or calendars are another great tool. Marking off each alcohol-free day can be incredibly satisfying. It's like giving yourself a little gold star for being awesome. These visual cues keep your motivation high and act as gentle nudges when needed.

Now, let's spice up those alcohol-free nights at home. Instead of reaching for a drink, why not try cooking new recipes together? Experimenting in the kitchen can be a fantastic bonding activity, and you get a delicious meal out of it. Transform your living room into a mini cinema with a movie marathon, popcorn, and cozy blankets. Or, dust off those board games and let the competition begin. Game nights can be a blast, filled with laughter and maybe a bit of friendly rivalry. These activities keep you entertained and reinforce that fun doesn't need to come in a glass.

Taking these steps turns your home into a supportive sanctuary where your goals feel achievable, and your resolve strengthens. It's about creating an environment that echoes your commitment to taking this dry month seriously but with a splash of creativity and a lot of enjoyment.

LEVERAGING DIGITAL TOOLS AND APPS FOR SUPPORT

In this tech-savvy world, your phone can be more than just a device for doom-scrolling through social media. It can be your sobriety coach, cheering you on with a range of apps designed to support your alcohol-free goals. Think of Sober Grid, which acts like a digital buddy offering community support. It's like having a pocket-sized pep squad where you can connect with others who are on this alcohol-free adventure. Then there's Drinkaware, an app that tracks those precious alcohol-free days. It's perfect for turning your dry month into a game of streaks, where each unbroken chain is a victory in itself. These apps keep you accountable and motivate you to keep going, even when the allure of a cool drink on a hot day seems almost irresistible.

The beauty of these digital tools lies in their ability to hold you accountable without the judgment of a stern-faced teacher. Daily reminders ping you with gentle nudges, akin to having a personal trainer for your sobriety. They remind you why you started and celebrate your milestones with virtual confetti. Imagine receiving a notification that you've saved a tidy sum by skipping cocktails—talk about motivation! These apps allow you to track your progress meticulously, turning your journey into a series of small victories that keep you motivated. Each day alcohol-free is another feather in your cap, bringing you closer to your goal. It's all about building a record of success, one day at a time.

Mindfulness and wellness apps are like the calm in the storm, offering guided meditation and exercises to help you navigate the choppy waters of craving and stress. Headspace, for example, provides guided meditation sessions that can help you find your zen when the world feels overwhelming. These apps teach you to breathe deeply, focus on the present, and find peace in everyday moments. Pair this with MyFitnessPal, which tracks your nutrition and exercise and has a holistic approach to wellness. Knowing what you're putting into your body and how it impacts your health can be eye-opening. These tools keep you grounded, showing you the benefits of mindfulness and healthy living.

Beyond apps, many online courses and webinars are available to deepen your understanding of sobriety. These resources offer insights into the benefits of going alcohol-free, delving into the science behind it. You can find webinars on stress management, offering strategies to keep your cool when life throws curveballs. Online courses cover topics from cognitive-behavioral techniques (CBT) to mindfulness practices, providing a toolkit for maintaining sobriety. It's like attending a virtual classroom, where you can learn at your own pace and apply new skills immediately. These educational resources empower you with knowledge, making you more resilient in facing challenges.

Take a Tech Break

Consider setting aside time each day to explore these digital resources. Create a schedule that includes using a sobriety app, engaging in a mindfulness session, and exploring an online course or webinar. This routine can reinforce your commitment and provide structure to your alcohol-free month. Keeping your digital toolbox ready ensures you have the support and guidance you need at your fingertips.

CELEBRATING MILESTONES WITH YOUR SUPPORT NETWORK

Imagine you're running a marathon. Every mile marker passed reminds you how far you've come, fueling your determination to reach the finish line. Celebrating milestones during Dry January works the same way. Acknowledging your progress, no matter how small, is crucial because it boosts motivation and reinforces the positive behaviors you're cultivating. Each day you go without a drink is another step towards a healthier you, and celebrating these achievements can be a powerful motivator. It's like giving yourself a high-five, reminding you that you're doing something incredible. These celebrations can be as simple as treating yourself to a favorite meal or as grand as planning a special outing. The important thing is to mark the occasion, pause, and say, "I did this."

So, how do you celebrate without reaching for the bubbly? Hosting a mocktail party is a fantastic option. Gather your friends, whip up some creative non-alcoholic concoctions, and toast to your success. It's fun to socialize and enjoy the moment without the morning-after regrets. Or maybe you prefer something more personal, like a day trip to a favorite hiking spot or a visit to a local art exhibit. Turning milestones into memorable experiences solidifies your achievement and enriches your life with new adventures. This approach shifts the focus from what you're avoiding to what you're gaining, emphasizing the joys of living entirely without alcohol.

Shared celebrations with your support network can create bonds that last long after the month is over. These moments become stories you'll tell for years to come, strengthening the ties that bind you. Imagine gathering with your tribe, reminiscing about the challenges and triumphs of the month while enjoying a delicious homemade feast. It's about creating a sense of community where everyone feels valued and part of something bigger than themselves. These shared experiences can be incredibly rewarding, fostering a sense of belonging and camaraderie that enriches your relationships.

Recognizing your achievements also comes with psychological perks that can't be overstated. Celebrating your wins—big or small—builds self-esteem. It's like giving yourself a gold star, boosting your confidence with each pat on the back. When you acknowledge your progress, you affirm your capability and resilience, which enhances your sense of accomplishment. This positive reinforcement can propel you forward, encouraging even bolder steps towards your goals. It's a cycle of success that feeds itself, creating a momentum that can carry you through future challenges with greater ease. By taking the time to celebrate, you're not just marking the end of a chapter; you're setting the stage for even greater achievements to come.

And so, with each milestone celebrated, remember that you're not just counting days; you're making every moment count. As you continue building this support network, think of it as a foundation for the healthier, more vibrant life you create. Now, onward to new adventures and discoveries!

4

NAVIGATING SOCIAL SITUATIONS

I magine you're at your cousin's wedding, where the open bar flows like Niagara Falls, and Aunt Marge is already three glasses in, ready to hit the dance floor. You're committed to Dry January, and the social pressure is as thick as the icing on the wedding cake. But fear not, because navigating social gatherings without a drink in hand doesn't have to feel like an episode of Survivor. In fact, with a little planning and a dash of creativity, you might find yourself having more fun than ever, all while dodging the dreaded hangover.

STRATEGIES FOR SOCIAL EVENTS AND PARTIES

Heading into any social event sans alcohol starts with solid pre-event planning. Picture yourself as a party ninja, stealthily setting personal boundaries and crafting an exit strategy that would make James Bond proud. Before you even leave the house, decide how you want the night to unfold. Set clear intentions about your boundaries, like how late you want to stay or how much socializing you're comfortable with. This mental prep can make all the difference. If the event is far from home and you anticipate an early night, arranging transportation ahead of time is key. Whether it's the trusty rideshare app like Uber or

Lift or a designated driver, having a plan means one less thing to worry about.

Let's talk about beverages. You wouldn't go to a potluck without bringing a dish, so why head to a party without your own non-alcoholic drink? Bring along your favorite non-alcoholic beer or a thermos filled with a homemade mocktail that's sure to impress. Not only does this ensure you have something tasty to sip on, but it also saves you from the dreaded solo cup of flat cola fate. Plus, you might spark some curiosity among fellow partygoers, turning your mocktail into the talk of the night. Remember, nothing says "I'm a responsible adult" like arriving with your own beverage.

Finding allies at the event can transform the experience from daunting to delightful. Seek out a friend who's also participating in Dry January or a family member who's in the know about your goals. Having someone in your corner can make all the difference. They can offer moral support, help steer conversations away from drink-related topics, and even join you in non-alcoholic solidarity. You'll be an unstoppable duo, navigating the party like seasoned pros.

When the DJ kicks up the tunes, dive into activities that don't revolve around drinking. Hit the dance floor with all the enthusiasm of a kid at a candy store, or jump into a game of charades with the same gusto. Engaging in these activities not only keeps you occupied but also shifts the focus from what's in your glass to the laughter and fun you're sharing. You might even find that your dance moves are smoother without the liquid courage or that you're the reigning champ of trivia night.

To keep the conversation flowing, dive into deep discussions beyond typical small talk. Ask open-ended questions, share stories, and really listen to what others have to say. You'll be surprised at the connections you can make when fully present and not distracted by the bar. These interactions can lead to meaningful conversations that leave a lasting impression long after the music fades and the party ends.

Party Prep Checklist

- Plan Your Boundaries: Decide how long to stay and what you're comfortable with.
- Bring Your Own Beverage: Pack a non-alcoholic drink you enjoy.
- Find Your Allies: Connect with friends or family who support your goals.
- Engage in Activities: Focus on games and dancing to stay entertained.
- Deepen Conversations: Foster connections through meaningful dialogue.
- With these strategies in your back pocket, you're ready to tackle any social situation that comes your way.

HOW TO POLITELY DECLINE ALCOHOL

Picture yourself at a lively dinner party, the room buzzing with chatter, and someone offers you a glass of wine. You're committed to staying dry this month, but how do you decline without sounding like a party pooper? Enter assertive communication, your best friend in these moments. A simple "No, thank you, I'm on a health kick right now" conveys your choice without inviting further questions. It's straightforward and lets others know your priorities without appearing preachy. Alternatively, try saying, "I'm not drinking tonight, but thanks for offering." This approach is equally polite and firm, setting your boundaries clearly.

A ready-made alternative reason can also be your ticket to a smooth decline. When someone offers you a drink, saying, "I'm driving tonight," or "I have an early morning tomorrow," provides a practical excuse that most people will respect. These responses are simple, relatable, and effective in deflecting pressure without making a big deal. They offer a quick way out of the situation, allowing you to continue enjoying the event without the burden of an unwanted drink.

Sometimes, a little humor can ease the tension and make saying no more comfortable. Picture yourself grinning and saying, "I'm trying to see if I can actually dance without liquid courage." It's lighthearted and can even spark a laugh, shifting the focus away from your drink choice and back to the fun of the evening. Using humor makes your decline feel less awkward and shows that you're still there to enjoy the moment, just without the booze. It can diffuse any lingering pressure and keep the mood upbeat.

Non-verbal cues are another powerful tool in your arsenal. Holding a non-alcoholic drink in hand can subtly communicate your choice without you having to say a word. It's like holding a shield of confidence, silently declaring your intentions. Coupled with a friendly smile and direct eye contact, your body language reinforces your decision. This approach shows you're comfortable with your choice and can often prevent further questioning from others. It's a quiet yet effective way to stand your ground.

Quick Comebacks

Sometimes, the most straightforward responses are the most effective. Here are a few quick comebacks to keep in your back pocket:

"I'm good with what I've got, thanks!"

"Just water for me tonight!"

"I'm on a drink break—cheers to that!"

By using these strategies, you'll find that declining a drink doesn't have to be a daunting task. It's about being comfortable with your choice, communicating it clearly, and maybe even having a little fun along the way.

HOSTING YOUR OWN ALCOHOL-FREE GATHERINGS

Planning an alcohol-free gathering can be as exhilarating as planning a getaway, minus the TSA lines and questionable airplane meals. The key to a successful event lies in engaging your guests with activities that make them forget they're not drinking. Think board game nights where Monopoly becomes a high-stakes showdown, and everyone's inner competitive spirit comes alive. Whether Scrabble or Catan, games offer a perfect icebreaker and keep everyone entertained. If board games aren't your style, consider hosting a cooking class or potluck. Invite your guests to showcase their culinary talents, turning your kitchen into a lively hub of tasty creations and laughter. There's something about chopping veggies together that brings people closer. The best part? Everyone gets to take home the recipe for the evening's culinary masterpiece, ensuring the fun doesn't stop when the party ends.

The ticket is to create a welcoming environment that feels as warm as a summer's day. Begin by setting a fun and relaxed atmosphere, perhaps with a playlist that has everyone humming along. Soft lighting, a few candles, or even a string of fairy lights can transform any room into a cozy haven. Think of it as setting the stage for the night's performance. As your guests arrive, greet them with a variety of non-alcoholic beverages that make their taste buds do a happy dance. From sparkling water with a twist of lime to more adventurous concoctions, having a range of options ensures everyone finds something they love. It's all about making them feel at home like they've just walked into their favorite café, where the barista knows their order by heart.

Speaking of beverages, what's an alcohol-free gathering without some delicious mocktails? With its refreshing mix of mint, lime, and soda, a Virgin Mojito is a crowd-pleaser that never disappoints. Or perhaps a Sparkling Cucumber Limeade, with its crisp and invigorating flavors, is more your style. These are simple to make but pack a punch in flavor, leaving guests impressed and reaching for refills. The beauty of these mocktails lies in their versatility, allowing you to get creative with garnishes like fresh fruit or herbs. It's like crafting a work of art in a glass that delights both the eyes and the palate.

The benefits of alcohol-free gatherings extend far beyond the absence of hangovers. Imagine waking up the next day feeling refreshed and ready to tackle the world instead of nursing a throbbing headache. This newfound clarity allows for more meaningful conversations where you're fully present and engaged. Without alcohol clouding judgment, interactions become genuine, and connections deepen. Guests leave feeling uplifted, having made memories that aren't hazy around the edges. It's a revelation, really, realizing that fun doesn't need to come with a side of regret. Instead, it comes with laughter, camaraderie, and perhaps a few new friendships.

Hosting an alcohol-free gathering is more than just an event; it's a celebration of life in its purest form, where every moment is savored, and every laugh is genuine. So go ahead, call some friends, and let the good times roll.

MANAGING SOCIAL ANXIETY WITHOUT ALCOHOL

Imagine walking into a crowded room, and suddenly, your heart feels like it's running a marathon. Social anxiety can really spoil the fun, making social interactions feel like climbing Everest in flip-flops. But here's the thing—alcohol isn't the only way to calm those nerves. Practicing mindfulness and grounding techniques can be your secret weapon. Start with some simple deep breathing exercises. Inhale slowly, hold and exhale—repeat until your heartbeat finds its rhythm. It's like hitting the reset button on your body's anxious autopilot. For a quick reality check, try the 5-4-3-2-1 grounding technique. Identify five things you can see, four you can touch, three you can hear, two you can smell, and one you can taste. It's a surefire way to anchor yourself in the present and remind your brain that everything's okay.

Preparation is your best friend when it comes to building confidence before social interactions. Think of it as studying for a test, but it is way more fun. Start by practicing small talk topics. Whether it's the latest Netflix series or the weather's quirky antics, having a few conversation starters tucked in your back pocket can ease the pressure. Visualizing positive outcomes is another powerful technique. Picture yourself mingling easily, laughing at jokes, and leaving with new friends. This mental rehearsal can make the real thing feel less daunting, like stepping into a scene you've already rehearsed a hundred times in your mind.

Finding support in anxiety resources can provide a comforting safety net. Consider joining an anxiety support group, where you'll meet others who get it and can offer tips that have worked for them. Something is reassuring about knowing you're not alone in this. For those digital-friendly moments, apps like Calm or Headspace can guide you through relaxation exercises, helping you unwind anytime, anywhere. They're like having a pocket-sized therapist, ready to remind you to breathe and find your happy place amidst the chaos. And don't forget, it's perfectly okay to lean on these resources whenever you need a little extra support.

Self-care is the cherry on top of your anxiety-busting routine. Before heading out to an event, indulge in a relaxing bath. Let the warm water melt away your worries, leaving you refreshed and ready to face the world. After the event, take a moment to journal about the experience. Reflect on what went well and what you'd like to improve next time. Writing it down can be cathartic, a way to release lingering tension and celebrate your successes, no matter how small. It's like conversing with yourself, offering insights and encouragement for future adventures.

Social anxiety doesn't have to steal the spotlight at your next gathering. With a little mindfulness, preparation, support, and self-care, you'll be ready to face any social situation confidently. Remember, you've got this—one breath, one step, one small talk topic at a time.

MOCKTAIL HOUR: FUN AND INCLUSIVE ALTERNATIVES

Envision your living room transformed into a vibrant oasis, the air filled with chatter and laughter, as guests mingle over colorful drinks that rival any cocktail. That's the magic of a well-organized mocktail hour, a gathering where the fun flows as freely as the non-alcoholic beverages. Start by sending out invitations that spark excitement, whether a quick text to your closest pals or a quirky digital invite complete with a hint of the tropical theme to come. The anticipation builds long before the first guest walks through the door, setting the stage for an unforgettable evening. With the right vibe in place, let's talk setup. The heart of your mocktail hour is the mocktail bar, a dazzling display of colors and flavors that invites guests to explore. Stock it with an array of mixers, fresh fruits, and garnishes, encouraging a hands-on approach to drink-making. It's like setting up a mini chemistry lab where the experiments are delicious, and the results are always satisfying. By having everything readily available, you empower your guests to become mixologists for the night, crafting drinks that are as unique as they are.

Sharing a variety of mocktail recipes caters to different tastes and adds an element of surprise to the evening. Consider offering a Tropical Pineapple Punch, a refreshing blend that transports your taste buds to a sunny beach with its tropical notes and vibrant hue. For those who prefer something a bit tangier, a Berry Lemonade Fizz could be the perfect concoction, combining the sweet and sour tang of berries with a fizzy finish that dances on the palate. These recipes are not only delightful but also simple to prepare, ensuring that you spend more time enjoying the party and less time playing bartender. With a drink in each hand, guests are ready to explore the festive atmosphere you've created.

Now, let's discuss décor. A festive atmosphere elevates any gathering, turning a simple event into a celebration. Imagine your space decked out in tropical or beach themes, with colorful glasses and creative garnishes that make every sip feel like a vacation. Think bright tablecloths, tiki torches, or even a sandcastle centerpiece if you're feeling adventurous. These elements don't just look great—they create an immersive experience that guests will love. Every detail, from the décor to the drinkware, contributes to the ambiance, making your mocktail hour a feast for the senses. It's about crafting an environment that encourages relaxation, conversation, and a whole lot of fun.

Engaging guests with interactive elements ensures that your mocktail hour is anything but ordinary. Consider a mocktail-making competition, where attendees get hands-on, crafting their signature drinks and vying for the title of best mixologist. Provide a selection of ingredients and let creativity run wild. Taste-testing and rating each creation adds a layer of friendly competition, with guests eager to sample the diverse array of concoctions. This activity entertains and fosters camaraderie as participants share tips and tricks, laugh over unexpected flavor combinations, and cheer for each other's successes. It's all about creating moments of joy and connection that linger long after the last glass is empty.

5

EMBRACING HEALTH AND WELLNESS

S o, you're finally diving into that novel you've been meaning to read, and suddenly, the words seem to jump off the page with newfound clarity. That's what abstaining from alcohol can do for your brain. It's like upgrading from a murky fishbowl to a pristine aquarium. Within just days of going alcohol-free, you'll likely experience a mental shift. It's as if someone switched on the lights upstairs, illuminating those cobwebbed corners of your mind. Tasks that once felt like Herculean chores become manageable, and you might even find yourself multitasking like a pro.

IMPROVEMENTS IN MENTAL CLARITY AND FOCUS

One of the most immediate benefits of cutting out alcohol is the boost in concentration. Whether you're crunching numbers at work or trying to keep up with the latest plot twists in your favorite TV series, you'll find your focus is sharper than ever. The fog lifts, revealing a world where details pop, and tasks flow seamlessly. The days of rereading the same paragraph five times because you got distracted by a squirrel outside your window are gone. Welcome to a world where your brain feels like it's running on premium fuel.

The long-term cognitive benefits are just as compelling. Sustained sobriety isn't just about today; it's an investment in your future. By keeping alcohol at bay, you're lowering your risk of cognitive decline and debilitating conditions like dementia. It's like giving your brain a protective shield against the ravages of time. Memory retention improves, helping you recall names, dates, and even where you left your keys. Think of it as a mental savings account, where the dividends are priceless memories and mental agility.

With mental clarity comes a surge in productivity and performance. Imagine breezing through your to-do list like a hot knife through butter. Achieving work-related goals becomes more efficient, and you might even find yourself with time to spare. That newfound clarity also enhances creativity and problem-solving skills. Suddenly, those eureka moments come with delightful frequency, and you find innovative solutions to challenges that once seemed insurmountable. It's like unlocking a hidden room in your brain, filled with untapped potential and bright ideas.

Self-Reflection: Your Mental Clarity Check

Take a moment to reflect on your own experience with mental clarity. Grab a journal and jot down how cutting back on alcohol has impacted your focus and productivity. Consider these questions:

- Have you noticed a change in your ability to concentrate on tasks?
- Are there areas of your life where you feel more creative or efficient?
- How has your memory improved since you began this journey?

This exercise can help you recognize and celebrate the improvements in your mental clarity and focus, motivating you to continue embracing a healthier lifestyle.

PHYSICAL HEALTH BENEFITS: SKIN, SLEEP, AND ENERGY LEVELS

Imagine waking up, glancing in the mirror, and noticing your skin looks like it's had a mini-makeover while you slept. That's the magic of quitting alcohol. Alcohol, despite its cheerful reputation, can wreak havoc on your skin. It's like that friend who overstays their welcome, leaving a mess behind. Without alcohol, your skin has a chance to heal. Acne and inflammation begin to fade, replaced by a natural glow that says, "I'm fresh and fabulous." Your skin's hydration improves, with elasticity bouncing back like a well-sprung trampoline. The result? A smooth, radiant complexion that practically screams, "Look at me, I'm thriving!"

Now, let's talk about the beauty of sleep. We're not just talking about any sleep, but the kind that has you waking up ready to conquer the world. Alcohol might lull you into dreamland, but it's notorious for disrupting the REM cycle, which is crucial for restful slumber. With alcohol out of the picture, your body enjoys uninterrupted sleep, letting you drift into deeper, more restorative phases. You wake up feeling refreshed, as if you've just spent the night in a five-star hotel bed instead of your trusty old mattress. Gone are the days of groggy mornings and caffeine-fueled starts. Instead, you greet the day with clarity and alertness, making every morning feel like the first day of spring.

Let's imagine you're running up a flight of stairs, and instead of feeling like you're scaling K2, you're bounding up with the energy of a gazelle. That's the boost giving up alcohol can provide. Without booze weighing you down, your energy levels soar. You find yourself more animated throughout the day, not just surviving, but thriving. Whether tackling a workout or simply playing with your kids, you've got the stamina to go the extra mile. This newfound vitality makes every task seem less daunting and more like a dance, with energy that flows effortlessly from one activity to the next.

Let me share a story about Lisa, who decided to cut out alcohol and found her skin, thanking her in ways she hadn't imagined. "I didn't realize how much alcohol was affecting my complexion until I stopped," she mentioned. Her skin cleared up, revealing a radiance she hadn't seen since her teenage years. Then there's Tom, who once relied on energy drinks to get through his day. After ditching alcohol, he noticed he no longer needed his afternoon caffeine fix. "It's like I flipped a switch," he said, marveling at his newfound energy and productivity. He even took up cycling, something he hadn't had the energy for in years.

So, what's the takeaway? Quitting alcohol doesn't just benefit your liver or wallet; it transforms your skin, revitalizes your sleep, and injects a dose of energy into your everyday life. It's not about deprivation; it's about discovering the vibrant, energetic you that's been waiting to break free. As you continue on this path, relish the changes you see and feel. Your skin, sleep, and energy levels are just the beginning of the incredible physical health benefits that await.

EMOTIONAL AND PSYCHOLOGICAL WELL-BEING

Imagine standing in the middle of a tornado of emotions, where mood swings and unexpected outbursts are the norm. Now, picture stepping out into calm, clear skies. That's the transition many experience when they cut back on alcohol. Alcohol, for all its promises of relaxation and fun, can actually act like a mischievous puppeteer, pulling at the strings of your emotions. It can amplify stress and make even the smallest challenges seem like monumental tasks. By reducing or eliminating alcohol, you can achieve greater emotional stability. Your emotions become more predictable, and you gain an enhanced ability to cope with stress. It's like switching from a rollercoaster to a serene gondola ride, where you're finally in control of your emotional landscape, not the other way around.

There's a strong connection between sobriety and the reduction of anxiety and depression. Alcohol can often act as a crutch, a temporary fix for deeper emotional issues. Over time, though, it can exacerbate these feelings, creating a cycle that's hard to break. By stepping away from alcohol, you give your mood a chance to regulate and stabilize.

It's akin to rebooting your system, allowing for improved emotional regulation and a brighter outlook. Without alcohol clouding your perception, you're free to experience life's ups and downs with clarity and resilience. You learn to rely less on alcohol as a coping mechanism, discovering healthier ways to manage stress and anxiety. It's a bit like upgrading from an old, clunky software to a sleek, efficient new version that runs smoothly and efficiently.

Sobriety also opens the door to enhanced self-awareness. When you're not using alcohol to numb or distract, you start to gain a better understanding of your emotions and triggers. It's like holding up a mirror and seeing yourself, truly seeing, perhaps for the first time. This newfound clarity allows you to reflect on personal growth, understanding what makes you tick and what makes you thrive. You begin to notice patterns and triggers that might have previously gone unnoticed, providing valuable insights into your behavior and emotions. These realizations can be enlightening, offering a roadmap to personal growth and emotional insight built on authenticity and self-love. It's a journey of self-discovery that can lead to profound changes in how you live and interact with the world.

Engaging in regular therapy or counseling can be tremendously beneficial to maintain this emotional and psychological well-being. It's like having a trusted guide to navigate the complexities of your mind. Therapy provides a safe space to explore your feelings and thoughts, offering tools and strategies to manage them effectively. Alongside professional support, practicing mindfulness and meditation can serve as powerful allies. These practices help you stay grounded, present, and connected to your emotions, like a gentle anchor in the stormy seas of life. They encourage you to pause, breathe, and reflect, fostering a sense of peace and stability that can be transformative. Building a strong support network is also invaluable. Surrounding yourself with friends, family, or support groups who understand and encourage your goals can create a foundation of strength and resilience. It's like weaving a safety net beneath you, ready to catch you when life throws you off balance. Together, these practices form a comprehensive approach to nurturing your emotional and psychological well-being, empowering you to live a life that's rich in peace, balance, and fulfillment.

INCORPORATING MINDFUL MOMENTS INTO YOUR DAY

Mindfulness, at its core, is about being present and fully engaged in the moment, a bit like savoring a perfectly ripe peach without worrying about the sticky juice dribbling down your chin. It's not just a trendy buzzword thrown around by yoga instructors; it's a powerful tool in maintaining sobriety. Think of it as the mental equivalent of hitting pause on your life's remote control. Mindfulness reduces stress and enhances emotional well-being by focusing on the here and now. When you're mindful, you're not replaying yesterday's dramas or preemptively stressing about tomorrow's challenges. You're right here, right now, and it's wonderfully freeing. It's like giving your brain a mini-vacation without needing travel insurance.

Incorporating mindfulness into your daily routine doesn't have to be complicated. Start your day with a short morning meditation session. Find a quiet corner, sit comfortably, and focus on your breathing. Even five minutes can set a positive tone for the day, much like a good breakfast sets up your metabolism. Throughout the day, practice mindful eating. Instead of scarfing down your lunch while checking emails, take a moment to appreciate the flavors and textures of your food. It's amazing how much more you enjoy a meal when you're not multitasking.

Mindful breathing exercises are another way to anchor yourself in the present. Three-part breathing, for example, involves inhaling deeply, holding the breath, and then exhaling slowly. It's like giving your lungs a gentle stretch. Then there's alternate nostril breathing, which sounds quirky but incredibly calming. By alternating between nostrils as you breathe, you balance your brain's left and right hemispheres. It's like a mini mind massage that leaves you feeling centered and refreshed.

Mindful movement takes mindfulness a step further, integrating the body and mind. Practices like yoga and Tai Chi offer a gentle way to move with intention, focusing on each movement and breath. It's like a dance between you and your awareness, where every step is deliberate and every breath is purposeful. Walking meditation is another fantastic option. Instead of rushing from point A to point B, walk slowly and mindfully, noticing the sensation of your feet touching the ground, the rhythm of your steps, and the world around you. It transforms a mundane activity into a rich sensory experience.

Mindfulness Exercise: Breathing Break

Try this simple breathing exercise whenever you feel stressed or overwhelmed. Find a comfortable seat, close your eyes, and take three deep breaths. Inhale deeply through your nose, hold for a moment, and exhale slowly through your mouth. With each breath, imagine stress leaving your body and calmness entering. Repeat this for a few minutes, and notice how your body and mind begin to relax. This practice can be done anytime, anywhere, offering a quick reset to keep you grounded throughout the day.

PRACTICING SELF-CARE WITHOUT ALCOHOL

You might picture bubble baths or a day at the spa, but let's expand that image. Self-care is a holistic practice, an all-encompassing approach to nurturing your entire being. It's about prioritizing your well-being in ways that truly nourish both body and mind. Alcohol might have been your go-to for unwinding, but there's a whole world of self-care practices that don't involve a drink. Imagine it as a personal wellness toolbox, minus the corkscrew. You're not just looking to unwind, you're looking to thrive. Your body deserves more than a temporary fix; it craves sustainable care that supports your health and happiness long-term.

Creating a relaxing evening routine is a great way to start. You come home after a long day, kick off your shoes, and settle into a comfy chair with a book or music that soothes your soul. Maybe you light a candle or brew a cup of herbal tea. The goal is to create a space that feels like a hug for your senses. Engaging in hobbies and interests can also be a form of self-care. Whether it's painting, gardening, or knitting, these activities allow you to lose yourself in a moment of creativity and joy. It's like giving your mind a mini-vacation, where stress fades, and fulfillment takes center stage.

Nourishing your body with healthy habits is crucial. Think of your body as a finely tuned instrument that needs the right fuel to perform its best. A balanced diet, rich in fruits, vegetables, lean proteins, and whole grains, is like a symphony of nutrients playing in perfect harmony. Staying hydrated with water and herbal teas ensures every cell in your body functions optimally. It's incredible how a simple glass of water can refresh your body and mind.

Emotional and mental self-care is equally important. Grab a journal and let the words flow. Journaling for self-reflection is like having a heart-to-heart with yourself, minus the awkward silences. It's a safe space to express feelings, explore thoughts, and set intentions. Setting boundaries and saying no is another powerful practice. It's about respecting your limits and prioritizing your needs. Remember, self-care isn't selfish; it's necessary. Saying no to others sometimes means saying yes to yourself, and that's perfectly okay. Boundaries act as a buffer, preserving your energy and keeping you grounded.

Start thinking of self-care as a lifestyle, not just a series of isolated acts. When you embrace self-care without alcohol, you give yourself the gift of clarity and peace. You're creating a foundation of wellness that supports you in every aspect of life. It's about being kind to yourself, understanding what makes you tick, and nurturing those needs. Self-care is the quiet confidence that comes from knowing you're taking care of yourself. It's the deep breath that releases tension, the laughter that bubbles up from a place of joy, and the serenity that follows a good night's sleep. So, as you navigate the landscape of self-care, remember that it's about finding what works for you and what makes you feel alive and content.

LONG-TERM HEALTH GOALS AND MAINTENANCE

Setting long-term health goals might seem daunting at first, like trying to eat a whole watermelon in one sitting. But breaking it down into manageable slices makes it a lot easier—and less messy. Start by identifying your health priorities. What do you want to achieve? Maybe it's shedding a few pounds, improving cardiovascular health, or just feeling more energetic. Once you have a clear vision, break these goals into smaller, actionable steps. For instance, if you aim to improve fitness, begin with a simple commitment to walk 10,000 steps a day or attend a weekly yoga class. Each small step is a building block, laying the foundation for your long-term success. Remember, Rome wasn't built in a day, and neither is a healthy lifestyle.

Maintaining healthy habits beyond Dry January requires more than sheer willpower. It's about creating a sustainable routine that fits seamlessly into your life. It is like finding the perfect pair of jeans—they should feel comfortable and look good. To do this, weave healthy habits into your daily routine, making them as natural as brushing your teeth. Regularly reassess and adjust your goals to keep them relevant and achievable. Life has a funny way of throwing curveballs; sometimes, your priorities might shift. That's okay. Flexibility is key. Maybe your goal of running three times a week becomes twice a week with a strength training session. It's not about being rigid; it's about maintaining momentum, even if the path changes slightly.

Celebrating milestones is an often overlooked but essential part of reaching your goals. It's like stopping to smell the roses on a long hike. Each milestone represents progress, and recognizing these achievements can boost motivation and encourage continued effort. Treat yourself to something special when you hit a target. It doesn't have to be extravagant—a new book, a day trip, or even a decadent dessert might do the trick. Reflecting on your progress also helps you see how far you've come and reinforces the positive changes you're making. Progress might be slow, but it's still progress. So, give yourself a pat on the back—literally, if you have to.

Building a supportive environment is crucial to maintaining these long-term health goals. Surround yourself with positive influences, whether that's friends who encourage your new habits or a community group that shares similar goals. Making healthy choices is easier when you're not doing it alone. Continue to seek support and resources that align with your objectives. This might mean joining a local fitness class or participating in online forums where you can share experiences and gain insights. Your environment should be a space where healthy habits are nurtured, not hindered. When you create a support network, you're not just building a safety net; you're constructing a trampoline that propels you forward.

As we wrap up this chapter, remember that setting and maintaining long-term health goals is an ongoing process. It's about finding what works for you and sticking with it. Each step, no matter how small, brings you closer to a healthier, happier self.

WE VALUE YOUR FEEDBACK!

If you're finding "Mocktails over Cocktails" helpful in managing your alcohol consumption, improving your health, or achieving a successful Dry month, please consider leaving a review on Amazon.

Your honest review can:

- Help others discover effective strategies for a healthier lifestyle.

- Inspire friends and family to embrace mindful living.

- Support our community in spreading the benefits of enjoying delicious mocktails.

Leaving a review is easy:

1. Scan the QR code below or visit the book's Amazon 'Write a customer review' page.

2. Share your thoughts and experiences.

Thank you for your support! Your feedback makes a big difference and helps us continue to promote wellness and mindful choices.

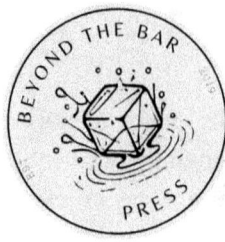

6

CRAVINGS AND WITHDRAWAL MANAGEMENT

I magine your brain as a bustling office, with neurotransmitters like dopamine playing the role of overly enthusiastic interns, running around delivering messages and ensuring everything feels just right. Now, alcohol is like the office party crasher, showing up uninvited and flooding the place with dopamine, turning the scene into a wild and euphoric shindig. But here's the catch: after the party, the interns are exhausted, their dopamine supplies depleted, leaving you feeling like a deflated balloon. This rollercoaster ride is what fuels alcohol cravings as your brain yearns for a return to that feel-good state. Over time, habitual drinking rewires your brain's chemistry, making it harder to experience pleasure without alcohol's presence. It's like your brain has gotten too used to the party and forgot how to have fun on its own. Understanding this cycle is crucial to managing cravings and taking back control.

UNDERSTANDING CRAVINGS AND TRIGGERS

Triggers are the sneaky little gremlins that set off cravings and can pop up when you least expect them. Social triggers are the most notorious, lurking at parties, bars, or even in the company of that one friend who always insists on "just one more drink." Emotional triggers are equally mischievous, striking when stress levels spike, or boredom creeps in. They know when you're vulnerable and pounce like a cat on a laser pointer. Situational triggers are those predictable routines, like the end-of-day ritual of pouring a glass of wine or the weekly trivia night at your local pub. These triggers can feel as ingrained as your morning coffee ritual, making them challenging to shake.

To outsmart these pesky triggers, you first need to identify them. Consider creating a trigger identification worksheet where you jot down when and where your cravings hit hardest. Was it at the office happy hour or after a stressful meeting? Reflective journaling can also help, allowing you to explore your thoughts and emotions around these moments. You can anticipate and prepare for your patterns, like a chess player thinking several moves ahead by tuning into your patterns.

Awareness is the superhero cape you didn't know you needed. Recognizing your triggers is the first step to managing them, giving you the power to respond rather than react. Increased self-awareness allows you to spot the gremlins before they wreak havoc, arming you with strategies to sidestep their mischief. Case studies abound with tales of success, like that of Jane, who managed her cravings by swapping her after-work drink with a brisk walk. Or Ben, who found solace in a new hobby whenever a trigger reared its head. These stories remind us that awareness and adaptability are key in this battle against cravings.

Cravings Trigger Tracker

To help you on this path, consider using a Cravings Trigger Tracker. Note the time, place, and situation each time a craving hits. Reflect on any patterns that arise, and brainstorm strategies to tackle them head-on. This simple exercise can be your secret weapon in winning the cravings game.

MINDFULNESS EXERCISES FOR CRAVINGS

Mindfulness is like that wise friend who always seems to have it all together, calmly sipping tea while the world buzzes around them. It's about being fully present in the moment, noticing your thoughts and feelings without judgment. This practice can change the game for managing cravings, as it helps you recognize them as temporary waves rather than insurmountable tsunamis. Numerous studies back this up, showing that mindfulness can reduce the intensity of cravings and improve emotional regulation. By focusing on the here and now, you're less likely to react impulsively—like diving headfirst into the cookie jar—or, in this case, reaching for a drink.

Let's start with the body scan meditation, a tool for tuning into your body like a radio dial to your favorite station. Find a quiet spot, close your eyes, and take a few deep breaths. Begin by focusing on your toes, noticing any sensations without trying to change them. Slowly move your attention through each part of your body, all the way to the top of your head. This exercise helps you recognize physical sensations that might accompany cravings, such as tension or restlessness. Next, try mindful breathing techniques by inhaling deeply through your nose, holding for a moment, and exhaling slowly through your mouth. This rhythmic breathing can calm the mind and reduce stress, making cravings feel less overwhelming. Lastly, the five senses exercise invites you to ground yourself by engaging all your senses—what you see, hear, taste, touch, and smell. It's like hitting the pause button on a busy day, bringing you back to the present with a sense of calm.

Consistency is critical with mindfulness, much like watering a plant regularly to see it thrive. Set up a daily mindfulness routine, carving out even a few minutes to practice each day. Apps like Headspace or Calm offer guided sessions, making it easy to sneak mindfulness into your schedule. Think of it like brushing your teeth—just a few minutes each day can make a world of difference. Over time, these practices can become second nature, providing you with tools to manage cravings and stress more effectively.

Real-life success stories abound, illustrating how mindfulness can transform lives. Take Emily, for example, who struggled with cravings during stressful workdays. By incorporating mindfulness into her routine, she reached for healthier coping mechanisms—like squeezing a stress ball or taking a short walk—rather than a drink. Her overall well-being improved, with greater emotional stability and self-aware-ness. Or consider Tom, who used mindfulness to navigate social events without succumbing to peer pressure. He discovered that being present in conversations made them more engaging, and he left gather-ings feeling energized rather than drained. These stories highlight the power of mindfulness as a tool for managing cravings and enhancing overall quality of life.

HEALTHY SNACK IDEAS TO CURB CRAVINGS

Let's chat about food. It's not just about filling your stomach; it's about keeping those pesky cravings at bay. The link between diet and crav-ings is as real as your grandma's secret cookie recipe. Keeping your blood sugar levels stable is like ensuring your smartphone has enough battery—it keeps you functional and less prone to sudden crashes. When your blood sugar dips, your body starts yelling for a quick fix, often in the form of sugar, caffeine, or alcohol. So, maintaining a steady stream of nutrient-rich foods can help manage those cravings and keep you on track. Foods that support brain health, like those rich in omega-3 fatty acids, are also great allies. They nourish your brain, keeping it balanced and less likely to send desperate signals for a dopamine boost.

Now, onto the fun part: snacks! Fresh fruit and vegetable sticks are your go-to. They're easy to prepare and packed with vitamins and fiber. Think crunchy carrot sticks, refreshing cucumber slices, or a sweet mix of berries. Pair them with a handful of nuts or seeds, and you've got a satisfying snack that packs a punch of healthy fats and protein. Greek yogurt with a drizzle of honey is another fantastic option. It's creamy, delicious, and provides protein to keep you full. And let's not forget about dark chocolate—yes, you read that right! A small piece can satisfy your sweet tooth without the sugar crash. It's rich in antioxidants and has just enough sweetness to give you a little lift without going overboard.

Let's spice things up with some simple recipes for those who enjoy a bit of culinary adventure. Avocado toast with a twist is always a winner. Mash up some ripe avocado, sprinkle with a dash of chili flakes, and top with sliced cherry tomatoes or bacon on whole-grain bread. It's as tasty as it is Instagram-worthy. Or try a smoothie bowl loaded with superfoods. Blend a banana, a handful of spinach, and some frozen berries. Pour it into a bowl and top with chia seeds, sliced almonds, and a sprinkle of granola for crunch. Whip up a homemade trail mix if you feel like a snack trailblazer. Combine your favorite nuts, seeds, dried fruits, and maybe a few dark chocolate chips for a delicious and portable treat.

Staying hydrated is another key player in the cravings game. Sometimes, when you think you're hungry, you're actually just thirsty. Drinking plenty of water throughout the day can help keep cravings at bay and support overall well-being. Herbal teas are also a great option, providing a warm, comforting beverage without any caffeine or sugar. Consider making a refreshing detox water with cucumber and mint. Slice a cucumber, add a few sprigs of mint, and let it steep in a jug of water. It's like a mini spa day in a glass, keeping you hydrated and your taste buds happy.

A balanced diet, rich in nutrients and hydration, is a formidable shield against cravings. It's about nourishing your body to keep it satisfied and less tempted by quick fixes. When you feel a craving coming on, reach for a healthy snack or a glass of water. It's a simple yet effective strategy to keep you on track and feeling your best.

DISTRACTION TECHNIQUES: KEEPING BUSY

Imagine cravings as nagging houseguests who overstay their welcome. Distraction is your secret weapon to show them the door politely. Keeping busy is about more than just filling time. It's strategically redirecting your focus to activities that engage your mind and body. This approach works because cravings love to latch onto idle minds. When immersed in an activity, your brain's attention shifts away from the craving, leaving it nowhere to settle. Think of it as giving your brain a delightful detour, keeping it too occupied to entertain unhelpful impulses. This psychological tactic is backed by the idea that our brains can only entirely focus on one thing at a time. So, the more you're engrossed in something positive, the less room there is for cravings to squeeze in.

Now, let's explore the colorful world of distraction activities. Physical activities are a fantastic way to channel energy while keeping cravings at bay. Walking offers a change of scenery and fresh air, while yoga provides physical and mental reprieve, stretching away tension and temptation. Creative pursuits like painting or writing can transport you to another realm where time seems to fly. Who knows, you might even discover a hidden talent for watercolors or poetry. Social activities are equally powerful. Sometimes, a simple call to a friend or joining a local club can lift your spirits and shoo away those pesky cravings. Sharing a laugh or two can work wonders, reminding you you're supported and connected.

Consider diving into a new hobby if you want to expand your horizons. Gardening is a meditative way to nurture life while soaking in the sun. Photography lets you capture the beauty in the world, focusing your attention on the present moment. Perhaps you're inclined to take up a new sport or fitness routine, something that gets your heart pumping and your mood lifted. These hobbies aren't just distractions. They're investments in yourself, enriching your life with new skills and experiences.

Incorporating these activities into your daily routine doesn't have to feel like a chore. Think of it as designing your personal schedule, peppered with moments of joy. Start by creating a daily schedule that includes dedicated slots for different activities. This structure provides predictability and a sense of purpose, helping you to look forward to each part of your day. It can be beneficial to set reminders for activity breaks. A gentle nudge to take a walk or pick up that paintbrush can make all the difference, ensuring you prioritize these moments of engagement amidst the hustle and bustle. It's about crafting a day filled with pockets of positivity, where cravings have little room to settle.

When cravings come knocking, you're not alone. You have a toolkit of distractions ready to deploy at a moment's notice. It's about reclaiming your time and energy, directing them towards uplifting and inspiring activities. So go ahead, explore that new hobby, call a friend, or take a stroll. It's about keeping busy in a way that fills your life with meaning and joy, leaving cravings with nowhere to hide.

COGNITIVE-BEHAVIORAL TECHNIQUES FOR CRAVINGS

Your mind is like a bustling city, with thoughts darting around like frantic drivers during rush hour. Cognitive-behavioral therapy (CBT) is here to play the role of the city planner, helping to organize this chaotic traffic of thoughts and behaviors, particularly when cravings come knocking. At its core, CBT operates on the principle that our thoughts, feelings, and behaviors are interconnected. By changing one, you can influence the others. It's like the ultimate life hack for your brain, offering a way to untangle the web of habit loops that keep you reaching for alcohol.

One of the shining stars of CBT is a technique known as thought-stopping. It's designed to help you hit the brakes when unhelpful cravings-related thoughts start zooming through your mind. Imagine a mental stop sign that pops up whenever a craving nudges its way in, urging you to pause and steer your thoughts in a healthier direction. Then there's cognitive restructuring, which is all about challenging and reframing those pesky, distorted thoughts. If you catch yourself thinking, "I can't enjoy a party without a drink," CBT encourages you to question that belief. Is it really true? Or is it just a deeply ingrained habit whispering in your ear?

Behavioral activation strategies are another handy tool in the CBT toolbox. These involve intentionally engaging in activities that boost your mood and distract from cravings. Instead of following the usual routine that might lead to drinking, you might decide to go for a run or tackle that DIY project you've been putting off. These activities not only fill the time but also help shift your mindset, reducing the power of cravings over your day-to-day life.

Challenging negative thoughts is at the heart of CBT. Think of cognitive distortions as those annoying pop-up ads on the internet, always trying to sell you something you don't need. One common distortion is black-and-white thinking, where situations are seen in extremes: you're either a roaring success or a complete failure. Developing positive affirmations can counteract these distortions. Instead of succumbing to "I slipped up, so I might as well give up," try adopting a more balanced perspective: "I had a setback, but I can get back on track." This shift can transform your internal dialogue from a harsh critic to a supportive friend.

Incorporating CBT techniques into your life can be like installing a new operating system for your brain, one that empowers you to navigate cravings with confidence. Whether you're practicing thought-stopping or restructuring your beliefs, CBT offers a roadmap to help you reclaim control and pave the way for a healthier, more balanced relationship with alcohol.

COPING WITH WITHDRAWAL SYMPTOMS

Withdrawal symptoms can feel like an uninvited guest crashing on your couch, refusing to budge. When you decide to put down the bottle, your body might throw a tantrum, so it's good to know what to expect. Let's talk about physical symptoms first. Headaches can sneak up on you like that persistent fly buzzing around your picnic. Nausea might join the party, too, making your stomach feel like it's doing the cha-cha. These discomforts are your body's way of recalibrating and adjusting to life without alcohol interference. On the psychological side, anxiety and irritability can take center stage. You might find yourself feeling jittery like you've had one too many espressos, or snapping at your roommate for breathing too loudly. It's all part of the process, though not exactly the fun part.

Now, let's arm you with practical strategies to manage these symptoms. Hydration is your new best friend. Drinking plenty of water helps flush out toxins and alleviate headaches. Pair that with a balanced diet rich in nutrients, giving your body the fuel it needs to heal. Gentle exercise can also work wonders. A brisk walk or stretching can release endorphins, lift your mood, and ease physical tension. Don't underestimate the power of relaxation techniques, either. A warm bath infused with calming aromatherapy oils can soothe your senses and offer a respite from discomfort. A little self-care goes a long way in navigating withdrawal.

Addressing the psychological aspect of withdrawal requires a bit of a toolkit. Breathing exercises are a lifesaver for managing anxiety. Try inhaling deeply through your nose, holding for a few seconds, and then exhaling slowly through your mouth. It's like hitting the reset button for your racing thoughts. Journaling can also be incredibly cathartic, providing an outlet for your emotions. Scribble down your feelings, fears, and frustrations, and watch as the page absorbs them like a sponge. Don't hesitate to reach out for support when things feel particularly overwhelming. Whether it's a friend who knows how to listen or a professional counselor, having someone to lean on can make all the difference.

If you find that withdrawal symptoms are more than just a minor inconvenience, consider seeking professional help. Severe symptoms might require medical supervision to ensure your safety. Don't hesitate to contact helplines or support groups, where trained professionals can guide you through the process. It's important to remember that you're not alone, and there's no shame in reaching out for help when you need it. Medical supervision can provide peace of mind and ensure that you're navigating withdrawal safely.

Navigating withdrawal symptoms is like weathering a storm; it can feel intense, but it won't last forever. Armed with the right strategies and support, you're better equipped to face the challenges head-on. As you move forward, you'll find that the storm gradually gives way to clearer skies, opening the door to a healthier, more balanced life. With each step, you're not just moving away from alcohol; you're moving towards a version of yourself that's stronger, more resilient, and ready to tackle whatever comes next.

7

FINANCIAL AND PERSONAL GROWTH BENEFITS

I magine you're on a treasure hunt, and instead of an old map with an "X" marking the spot, your map is a series of receipts and bank statements revealing where your money has been mysteriously disappearing. Spoiler alert: a lot of it ends up at the local bar! But now, armed with the decision to cut back on alcohol, you're about to discover a hidden pile of savings that could fund your dreams, whether that's a trip to the Bahamas or that fancy espresso machine you've been eyeing. The key to unlocking this treasure is tracking your financial savings—because what's the point of saving money if you can't see just how much you're saving?

TRACKING YOUR FINANCIAL SAVINGS

Let's start by visualizing the impact of reduced spending. You know that dopamine rush when you find a $20 bill in your jeans pocket? Imagine that feeling on steroids when you realize how much you're saving by skipping those after-work drinks. Tracking these savings is crucial, not just for the feel-good factor, but to keep you motivated. When you see those numbers adding up, it's like watching your piggy bank get chubbier by the week. You become more committed to sticking with your goals because the results are tangible.

Setting up a tracking system doesn't have to be a chore. Thanks to modern technology, there are apps designed to make the process as painless as possible. The Reframe App, for example, helps you cut back on drinking and shows you exactly how much cash you're banking in the process. Creating a simple spreadsheet is a great alternative for those who like to get hands-on. List your typical monthly alcohol expenditure, and subtract your new spending habits. Voila! You've got a visual representation of your progress. It's like a financial Fitbit for your sobriety goals.

Now, into the math. Monthly and annual calculations can be surprisingly fun when they're in your favor. Start by comparing your past spending habits with your current ones. Include related expenses often accompanying drinking, like late-night takeout or those regrettable Uber rides home. Add it all up and get a clear picture of what you've managed to save. Seeing these figures in black and white can be a real eye-opener. Maybe those savings will cover that weekend getaway, or perhaps they'll go towards paying off that lingering credit card debt. The possibilities are endless.

Reviewing and adjusting your tracking system regularly is essential. Think of it like tuning up a car—you must keep everything running smoothly. By identifying patterns and trends in your spending, you can make informed decisions about where to tighten the belt or allow a little wiggle room. Maybe you notice that your spending spikes during social events, prompting you to plan ahead and bring your own non-alcoholic drinks. Adjustments ensure your system remains accurate and reflects your true financial picture.

REALLOCATING YOUR ALCOHOL BUDGET

Let's say you've managed to save a tidy little sum by cutting back on those evening cocktails and weekend bar hops. Now, you're standing at the metaphorical crossroads of decision-making, pondering where to direct this newfound wealth. The first step? Identifying all those sneaky little expenses where alcohol used to gobble up your cash. Dining out is a prime suspect. It's not just the drinks themselves but the marked-up prices that restaurants slap on them. By choosing water over wine, you can significantly slash your dining bills. The same goes for entertainment and social activities. Concerts, sports events, and theater outings often have alcohol as a central component. Opting for non-alcoholic beverages or skipping the bar line altogether means more money stays in your pocket.

With these savings in sight, it's time to craft a reallocation plan. Think of it as a budget makeover, where you set new financial priorities that better align with your goals. Start by taking a good, hard look at your current spending habits. Are there areas that could use a little love, like that neglected gym membership or an online course you've been eyeing? Allocate your funds to different categories that reflect your values and interests. This could be anything from health and wellness to personal development or even a fun fund for spontaneous adventures. By consciously directing your money, you take control of your finances and ensure that every dollar is working towards something meaningful.

Speaking of meaningful, consider investing your saved cash in activities that enrich your life. Educational courses and workshops are another fantastic option. Whether it's learning a new language, picking up a musical instrument, or diving into coding, these experiences broaden your horizons and add value to your life. Investing in yourself is always a win, and with the money saved from skipping those drinks, you can afford to explore new passions and skills. Consider attending a personal development seminar, those events where motivational speakers have you on your feet, clapping and nodding in agreement. The insights gained can be life-changing, equipping you with tools to tackle challenges head-on. Or perhaps it's time to enroll in online courses. Whether it's coding, public speaking, or culinary arts, each course adds a new feather to your cap, enhancing your skill set and broadening your horizons. It's like upgrading your personal operating system, one course at a time.

While you're at it, why not build a rainy-day fund? Setting up an emergency savings account is a smart move that provides peace of mind. Start by setting up automatic monthly transfers from your checking account to your savings account. Even a small amount can add up over time and act as a financial cushion when unexpected expenses arise. Establishing savings goals, like reaching a specific amount by the end of the year, can keep you motivated and focused. It's all about creating a safety net that allows you to handle life's curveballs without the stress of financial strain.

INVESTING IN NEW INTERESTS AND HOBBIES

You are now standing at the intersection of newfound financial freedom, your savings from skipping those happy-hour cocktails burning a hole in your pocket. What better time to explore new interests and hobbies? Maybe you've always wanted to try your hand at tennis, but the thought of investing in lessons seemed daunting. Now, with extra savings, you can finally swing that racket and maybe even channel your inner Serena Williams. Or perhaps you've been eyeing the dusty guitar in the corner, longing to strum like a rock star in your living room. Whether it's a new sport or learning an instrument, diving into these pursuits can be a thrilling adventure, sparking joy and maybe even surprising talents you never knew you had.

Creativity and self-expression are equally rewarding avenues for investment. Have you ever wanted to paint a masterpiece or craft a ceramic mug that's uniquely yours? Joining an art or craft class might be the ticket. It's not just about the end product; it's the process of creation that soothes the soul. Writing workshops or clubs offer similar fulfillment. Whether penning the next great novel or just pouring your thoughts into a journal, writing is a powerful form of self-expression, allowing you to explore and articulate your innermost thoughts and dreams. These creative pursuits aren't just hobbies; they're therapeutic outlets that enrich your life in countless ways.

Now, let's focus on building lasting habits through these personal investments. Setting long-term goals for skill mastery can be your guiding star. Imagine yourself six months down the line, no longer fumbling through guitar chords but strumming them with confidence. Or picture yourself crafting words with ease, your writing flowing effortlessly. Tracking progress is vital. Keep a journal or a visual chart to mark milestones. Celebrate each achievement, whether it's mastering a new chord or completing a chapter of your book. Celebrating these wins reinforces your commitment and motivates you to keep pushing the boundaries of your capabilities.

These investments are more than just pastimes; they're stepping stones to a richer, more fulfilling life. You're nurturing your growth and expanding your horizons by channeling your resources into personal development and hobbies. So go ahead; let your curiosity guide you. Whether you're hitting the tennis courts, creating art, or mastering a new skill, each step you take is a testament to your dedication to becoming the best version of yourself.

THE LONG-TERM FINANCIAL IMPACT OF SOBRIETY

Imagine standing at the precipice of financial freedom; all it took was saying "no" to that extra round of drinks. Long-term sobriety isn't just about feeling better; it's like watching your bank account go on a slow but steady diet, shedding unnecessary expenses in favor of healthy savings. Over the years, the cumulative savings from not indulging in alcohol can be staggering. Let's say you save $100 a month by cutting out those weekly bar trips. That's $1,200 a year. Now stretch that over a decade, and you're looking at $12,000! Compare that to other investments, like stocks or bonds, and you'll see that the decision to stay sober can rival some of your smartest financial moves. It's like finding a golden goose in your budget.

Opportunity costs are another financial kicker. By not spending on alcohol, you free up cash for investments that actually appreciate over time. Consider putting that saved money into stocks or mutual funds. These are investments that work for you, growing over the years and potentially providing a nest egg for the future. Perhaps you're dreaming of owning your own home. Those savings could be the start of a down payment, turning your dream into reality sooner than you think. Sobriety doesn't just save; it opens doors to opportunities that might have been financially out of reach. This shift from spending to investing is like swapping a leaky bucket for a sturdy, dependable one.

Then there's the thorny issue of debt. Those savings from sobriety can be the key to paying off debts. Imagine the relief of watching your credit card balances dwindle as saved funds are redirected to tackle outstanding bills. It's like using a battering ram to knock down the high walls of interest charges. Student loans, lingering from college days, can also be reduced. Every dollar that doesn't go into a cocktail can chip away at those balances, bringing you closer to financial independence. You're not just saving money but reclaiming your financial freedom, one sober decision at a time.

Building financial security is perhaps the most profound impact of staying sober. It's not just about having money in the bank; it's about creating a safety net that allows you to weather life's storms. Consider increasing your retirement savings. Those funds you used to spend on drinks could bolster your 401(k) or IRA, ensuring a comfortable future. Think about establishing a robust emergency fund. Life is unpredictable, and having a financial cushion can provide peace of mind, allowing you to handle unexpected expenses without stress. It's about creating a solid foundation, a fortress of financial stability that stands firm, ready to support you no matter what challenges arise. Sobriety is a personal health choice and a strategic financial move that pays dividends in ways you might never have imagined.

BUILDING CONFIDENCE THROUGH PERSONAL GROWTH

Imagine waking up one day and discovering that you are thriving rather than merely existing. That's the magic that happens when financial savings start to translate into increased confidence. It's like suddenly realizing you have a superpower nobody told you about. With each dollar saved you feel a little more in control, as if you've finally found the remote to the chaos that was your financial life. Knowing you can make choices that lead to economic stability is empowering. That empowerment is the kind of confidence booster that makes you walk a little taller. It's not just about the money; it's about the self-efficacy that comes from achieving your goals and proving to yourself that you can set your mind to something and see it through.

Personal growth goals are a natural extension of this newfound confidence. Think about what skills or competencies you've always wanted to develop. Maybe it's something career-related, like mastering a new software or learning a second language. Or perhaps it's more personal, like becoming a better cook or honing your public speaking skills. Whatever it is, setting goals that align with your financial savings can propel you forward. Exploring educational opportunities can be part of this growth. Enroll in that online course or attend a seminar that piques your interest. These investments in yourself can open doors not just in your career but also in your personal life. They're not just about adding lines to your resume; they're about becoming more well-rounded and confident.

Make sure to celebrate achievements along the way. It's like taking a pit stop on a long road trip to admire the scenery. Acknowledge the milestones you've reached, whether it's saving your first thousand dollars or completing a challenging course. Reward yourself in ways that matter, perhaps with an experience rather than a thing. Maybe it's a weekend getaway to recharge or a new book that promises adventure and inspiration. These rewards serve as reminders of your hard work and dedication, reinforcing the positive behaviors that got you there. They're not just treats; they're acknowledgments of your progress and motivation to keep pushing forward.

Maintaining momentum is the secret sauce to continuous improvement. Regularly reassess your goals and progress. Are you still on track? Do your goals still excite and challenge you? If not, it might be time to shake things up. Seek new challenges that reignite your passion for growth. This could mean setting a higher savings target or diving into a completely new hobby. It's about keeping the flame alive and ensuring you're always moving forward, avoiding the complacency that can come from resting on your laurels. Continuous growth isn't a destination; it's an ongoing process, a commitment to bettering yourself bit by bit, day by day.

As you build confidence through these avenues, remember that each step forward is a testament to your resilience and determination. The connection between financial savings and personal growth isn't just a theory—it's a tangible cycle that reinforces itself. You're saving money and investing in a more confident, capable you. With each achievement, you're not just ticking boxes but crafting a narrative of success and empowerment. It's the kind of growth that changes you and influences those around you. And as you look ahead, the possibilities are as exciting as they are endless.

8

MOCKTAILS AND NON-ALCOHOLIC ALTERNATIVES

Y ou're at a party, and the host asks, "What'll you have?" Instead of the usual, you opt for something different—a mocktail. Now, before you roll your eyes, let's take a little trip down memory lane. The term "mocktail" isn't some new-age trend. It's been around since 1916, a nod to the roots of non-alcoholic concoctions, or "temperance drinks," which were popular even before Prohibition. Bartenders back then were creative wizards whipping up delightful non-alcoholic versions of popular cocktails. Fast forward to today, and mocktails have evolved into a complex art form, thanks to mixologists who wield syrups, juices, and spices like culinary artists, creating anything but dull drinks.

THE ART OF MAKING MOCKTAILS

The art of making mocktails isn't just about throwing some juice in a glass with a splash of soda. It's a craft, much like painting or sculpting, but with liquids. Mastering this art involves a few basic techniques that can elevate your mocktail game. Shaking, stirring, and blending are the holy trinity of mixology. Shaking a mocktail with ice chills it quickly, melding flavors together. Stirring is ideal for drinks with clear ingredients, keeping them crisp and clean. Blending, meanwhile, is perfect for frosty, textured drinks that feel like a tropical escape. Presentation is the cherry on top. A well-garnished drink with a sprig of mint or a citrus twist turns a simple mocktail into a visual delight.

Balance is the secret ingredient in any great mocktail. It's about finding that sweet spot where flavors meld into perfection. Think sweet, sour, bitter, and umami—a symphony of tastes that work in harmony. Too much sweet, and the drink feels cloying; too tart, and it puckers your lips. It's like a dance, where each flavor takes its turn in the spotlight without stepping on anyone else's toes. Achieving this balance is the hallmark of a skilled mixologist, even when the spirits are non-alcoholic.

To create these masterpieces at home, you'll need some essential tools. Start with a good shaker and strainer to craft the perfect mocktail. A muddler is crucial for those mojito-style drinks, gently releasing the aroma of fresh herbs. Glassware, like the elegant Collins or the classic Old Fashioned glass, can transform the drinking experience. A measuring jigger ensures precision because, in the world of mocktails, a little too much or too little can make all the difference.

Now, let's stock that bar. Start with fresh fruits and vegetables. Citrus fruits—lemons, limes, oranges—are the backbone of countless beverages. Berries and tropical fruits like pineapples and mangoes bring a refreshing twist. Herbs and spices like mint, basil, and rosemary add depth, while spices like cinnamon and ginger provide warmth. Sweeteners like simple syrup, honey, agave nectar, and maple syrup offer varying levels of sweetness and complexity. Non-alcoholic spirits and mixers, like Seedlip™ or a good ginger beer, give depth and character to your creations.

Quality ingredients are paramount. Opt for organic fruits and herbs when possible. They may be pricier, but the flavor payoff is worth it. Artisan syrups and mixers add sophistication and nuance, elevating your mocktails from simple refreshments to gourmet experiences. Throw in some exotic ingredients like passion fruit or specialty bitters for a touch of the unexpected. These unique elements can turn a standard mocktail into something extraordinary, offering a taste adventure with every sip.

When it comes to storing ingredients, keep herbs fresh by wrapping them in a damp paper towel and storing them in the fridge. Properly cut and juice fruits to maximize flavor and minimize waste. Freshness is key, so use ingredients promptly to ensure your mocktails always taste their best. With these tips and tricks, you're well on your way to becoming a mocktail maestro.

STOCKING YOUR MOCKTAIL BAR

Essential Ingredients and Tools Checklist for Your Mocktail/Cocktail Bar

Creating a well-stocked mocktail and cocktail bar involves selecting a combination of essential tools, versatile ingredients, and unique elements that can elevate your drink creations. This comprehensive checklist is divided into categories to ensure you have everything you need to craft both classic favorites and innovative beverages.

1. Essential Tools and Equipment

Bar Tools:

- **Shaker:** Boston shaker (two-piece) or Cobbler shaker (three-piece) for mixing drinks.
- **Mixing Glass:** For stirring cocktails that don't require shaking.
- **Bar Spoon:** Long-handled spoon for stirring and layering drinks.
- **Muddler:** For crushing herbs, fruits, and spices to release flavors.
- **Jigger:** Measuring tool (typically 1 oz and 2 oz) for precise ingredient portions.
- **Strainer:** Hawthorne and fine mesh strainers to remove solids from shaken or stirred drinks.
- **Citrus Juicer:** Manual or electric juicer for fresh juice extraction.

- **Bottle Opener & Corkscrew:** Essential for opening beer, wine, and bottled mixers.
- **Ice Tools:** Ice scoop, ice tongs, and ice molds (crushed and cubed) for various drink needs.
- **Peeler:** For creating citrus twists and garnishes.

Glassware:

- **Highball Glasses:** For tall, mixed drinks like Mojitos and Spritzers.
- **Rocks Glasses (Old Fashioned):** For short drinks served over ice.
- **Martini Glasses:** For elegant cocktails and mocktails.
- **Coupe Glasses:** For classic cocktails like Manhattans and modern presentations.
- **Mason Jars:** Versatile for casual and rustic drink presentations.
- **Flute Glasses:** For sparkling beverages and celebratory drinks.
- **Shot Glasses:** For measuring and serving spirits.

Additional Equipment:

- **Blender:** For frozen cocktails and smoothies.
- **Juice Squeezer:** Manual squeezer for fresh citrus juice.
- **Speed Rack:** For organizing frequently used bottles within easy reach.
- **Bar Mat:** Protects surfaces and catches spills.
- **Cutting Board and Knife Set:** For preparing fresh ingredients and garnishes.
- **Glass Rimmer:** For adding salt, sugar, or other coatings to glass rims.
- **Storage Containers:** Airtight containers for storing ingredients and garnishes.

2. Essential Ingredients

Non-Alcoholic Bases:

- **Sparkling Water/Soda:** Adds fizz and lightness to mocktails.
- **Tonic Water:** Essential for non-alcoholic Gin & Tonics and other spritzers.
- **Coconut Water:** Adds a tropical twist and hydrates.
- **Non-Alcoholic Spirits:** Provides complexity without the alcohol, such as Seedlip or Ritual Zero Proof.

Mixers and Juices:

- **Fresh Citrus Juices:** Lemon, lime, and orange for brightness and acidity.
- **Pineapple Juice:** Adds sweetness and tropical flavor.
- **Cranberry Juice:** For tartness and vibrant color.
- **Ginger Beer/Ale:** Spicy and effervescent for Mule-inspired drinks.
- **Simple Syrup:** Basic sweetener made from sugar and water.
- **Honey Syrup:** For a richer, floral sweetness.
- **Grenadine:** Adds sweetness and a beautiful red hue.
- **Bitters:** Aromatic bitters like Angostura for depth and complexity.

Syrups and Flavorings:

- **Agave Nectar:** Natural sweetener, especially for Margarita-style drinks.
- **Orgeat Syrup:** Almond-flavored syrup for Mai Tais and other exotic cocktails.
- **Fruit Purees:** Such as mango, strawberry, or raspberry for added texture and flavor.
- **Herbal Infusions:** Rosemary, thyme, or basil syrups for unique herbal notes.
- **Flavored Extracts:** Vanilla, almond, or coconut for subtle enhancements.

3. Fresh Ingredients and Garnishes

Fruits:

- **Citrus Fruits:** Lemons, limes, oranges, and grapefruits for zest, juice, and slices.
- **Berries:** Strawberries, blueberries, raspberries, and blackberries for muddling and garnishes.
- **Tropical Fruits:** Pineapple, mango, and kiwi for vibrant flavors.
- **Apples and Pears:** Sliced for garnishes and added sweetness.

Vegetables and Herbs:

- **Mint Leaves:** Essential for Mojitos and other refreshing drinks.
- **Basil:** Adds an aromatic touch to savory and sweet cocktails.
- **Cucumber Slices:** For a crisp, clean flavor in drinks like Gin Fizz.
- **Celery Sticks:** For savory garnishes and Bloody Marys.

Garnishes:

- **Olives and Cocktail Onions:** For classic martinis and Gibson cocktails.
- **Cherries:** Maraschino or brandied cherries for sweet finishes.
- **Citrus Twists and Wheels:** For elegant and flavorful garnishes.
- **Sugar and Salt Rims:** Enhances flavor profiles of certain drinks like Margaritas or Daiquiris.
- **Edible Flowers:** Adds a sophisticated and decorative touch.
- **Spices:** Cinnamon sticks, star anise, or nutmeg for aromatic finishes.

4. Unique and Specialty Ingredients

Exotic and Artisanal Items:

- **Shrubs:** Vinegar-based syrups that add tanginess and complexity.
- **Tamarind Paste:** For a sour and slightly sweet flavor in innovative drinks.
- **Matcha Powder:** For a vibrant color and earthy taste in mocktails.
- **Activated Charcoal:** For striking visual appeal and detoxifying properties.
- **Hibiscus Syrup:** Adds floral notes and a rich color to beverages.

Specialty Spirits and Non-Alcoholic Alternatives:

- **Non-Alcoholic Wines and Beers:** Expands options for diverse mocktail offerings.
- **Flavored Bitters:** Orange or chocolate bitters provide unique flavor layers.

Superfoods and Functional Ingredients:

- **Chia Seeds:** Added texture and nutrition in healthy mocktails.
- **Turmeric:** Adds color and anti-inflammatory benefits.
- **Coconut Cream:** For rich, creamy textures in tropical drinks.
- **Aloe Vera Juice:** For a soothing and hydrating element.

Infused Ingredients:

- **Homemade Infused Syrups:** Such as lavender simple syrup or jalapeño agave.
- **Infused Waters:** Cucumber-mint or citrus-berry infusions for enhanced hydration.
- **Tea Bases:** Green, black, or herbal teas for depth and flavor.

By following this detailed checklist, you'll be well-equipped to set up a mocktail bar that caters to a wide range of tastes and occasions, ensuring that every drink you create is delightful and memorable.

MOCKTAIL RECIPES TO TRY

Imagine you're craving the refreshing zest of a mojito but without the buzz. Enter the **Virgin Mojito**, a classic reimagined with all the minty goodness and tangy lime, minus the rum. Muddle fresh mint leaves with simple syrup, add lime juice, and top with soda water. It's the kind of drink that makes you feel like you're on a tropical getaway, even if you're just lounging in your backyard. Then there's the **Non-Alcoholic Margarita**, perfect for those who love the salty-sweet dance of lime and agave. Mix lime juice, orange juice, and a splash of agave syrup, served over ice with a salted rim. It's a fiesta in a glass, no tequila required!

For those days when you want something light and breezy, reach for a **Berry Bliss Spritzer**. This concoction combines mixed berries, a hint of lemon juice, and bubbly soda water, creating a drink that sparkles as much as it refreshes. Or try the **Tropical Mango Cooler**, blending ripe mango puree with a splash of coconut water and a squeeze of lime. It's like sipping sunshine, perfect for a warm day when you need a little cooling off.

When you're in the mood for something with a little more depth, herbal and spiced mocktails are your ticket. **Rosemary Lemonade** is a delightful twist on a classic, with rosemary sprigs infusing lemon juice and honey for a refreshing and sophisticated drink. Then there's the **Ginger Peach Fizz**, a blend of peach puree, ginger syrup, and soda water. It's a little sweet, a little spicy, and entirely satisfying.

Craving something rich and creamy? Enter the **Coconut Pineapple Smoothie**. Blend coconut milk with fresh pineapple chunks for an indulgent and healthy tropical delight. For a dessert in a glass, try the **Chocolate Mint Delight**. Mix chocolate syrup with milk and a dash of mint extract, then serve over ice for a cool, creamy treat. It's like enjoying a chocolate mint candy bar without the sugar rush.

Non-Alcoholic Beverages for Every Occasion

Brunch without a Bloody Mary is like pancakes without syrup—something feels off. Enter the **Virgin Bloody Mary**, a spicy staple that pairs perfectly with eggs benedict or avocado toast. It's a robust blend of tomato juice, a dash of Worcestershire sauce, a hint of hot sauce, and a squeeze of lemon. Garnish with celery and olives, and you've got a zesty, savory drink that holds its own at any brunch table. And if you're in the mood for something a bit lighter, try a **Citrus Sunrise Mimosa**. Combine orange juice with a splash of sparkling water and a hint of grenadine for a sunrise of flavors without the champagne headache. It's brunch in a glass, with all the sunshine and none of the clouds.

When dinner parties roll around and the clinking of glasses fills the air, you might want something a bit more sophisticated. The **Cucumber Basil Cooler** is a refreshing, elegant choice. Think crisp cucumber slices muddled with fresh basil, topped with sparkling water for a drink that whispers sophistication. Its light, herbal notes make it a perfect companion to a summer salad or grilled fish. For a pop of color and flavor, the **Pomegranate Sparkler** is your go-to. Mix pomegranate juice with a splash of lime and top with soda water. This drink dazzles with its deep red hue and tart, sweet taste, making it an ideal match for a stylish soiree.

Celebrations call for something that feels as festive as the occasion. The **Sparkling Grape Punch,** with its bubbly effervescence and sweet-tart grape flavor, is perfect for toasting without the alcohol. Mix grape juice with a splash of sparkling water and a hint of lemon for a drink that's as celebratory as a fireworks display. Or perhaps you're hosting a holiday gathering; the **Cranberry Apple Cider** will stand out. It's a warm blend of cranberry juice, apple cider, and spices like cinnamon and cloves, perfect for cozy evenings with friends.

After a long day, relaxation is necessary, and your drink should reflect that. **Lavender Chamomile Tea** is like a warm hug in a mug, with calming chamomile and soothing lavender coming together to ease your mind. Perfect for sipping before bed or during a quiet afternoon.

The Honey Lemon Ginger Tonic is a fantastic choice if you prefer something with a bit of zing. This drink combines honey, fresh ginger, and lemon for an invigorating and comforting tonic. It's the kind of drink that warms you from the inside out, bringing a sense of tranquility with every sip.

Mocktail Recipes to Try at Home

Imagine yourself in a cozy kitchen, the heart of your home, ready to whip up some delightful mocktails that promise to dazzle your taste buds while keeping your sobriety intact.

First up is the **Berry Lemonade Fizz**, a fruity concoction perfect for those who crave a little zing. Get some mixed berries—strawberries, raspberries, blueberries—and mash them slightly. Mix with lemon juice and a splash of simple syrup, then pour over ice. Top it off with club soda, and watch as the bubbles dance. This drink is like a burst of summer, regardless of the season. For a tropical twist, the **Tropical Mango Punch** is your go-to. Blend ripe mango chunks with pineapple juice and a hint of coconut milk. Serve over ice with a lime wedge. Each sip is like a mini-vacation, offering a taste of the tropics.

A few tips can go a long way to perfect these recipes. Adjusting sweetness might be needed; taste as you go and tweak the syrup to your liking. Presentation matters, too. Garnish with a twist of citrus or a handful of berries to make your drinks look as good as they taste. High-quality images can inspire your creations, showing you what to aim for and sparking ideas for your own variations. Mocktails are as much about creativity and fun as they are about flavor, so don't hesitate to experiment.

Seasonal Mocktails for Every Occasion

Consider mocktails as the ever-changing wardrobe of your beverage world, adapting to each season with flair. The beauty of using seasonal ingredients lies in their freshness and vibrant flavors that can elevate your mocktail game. In summer, think juicy watermelons mingling with mint for a **Watermelon Mint Cooler** that's as refreshing as a dip in the pool. Meanwhile, fall brings a cascade of apples, perfect for a

Spiced Apple Cider Punch that warms you from the inside out. Come winter, cranberries and spices swirl together in a **Cranberry Spice Fizz**, reminiscent of cozy nights by the fire. When spring arrives, strawberries and basil pair up in a **Strawberry Basil Refresher**, offering a taste of the season's renewal.

Seasonal garnishes are the finishing touch. Fresh mint sprigs complement summer's coolers, while cinnamon sticks add a touch of warmth to fall and winter concoctions. These small details enhance flavor and make your drinks visually appealing, adding an extra layer of enjoyment. Hosting a seasonal mocktail party can be a delightful way to showcase these creations. Decorate with seasonal themes—think sunflowers and seashells in summer or pumpkins and leaves in autumn. Pair the drinks with dishes that echo the season's bounty, like a crisp summer salad with the Watermelon Mint Cooler or a hearty stew with the Spiced Apple Cider Punch. Encourage guests to bring a dish that complements the mocktail of their choice, turning your gathering into a culinary celebration.

When planning these themed gatherings, consider the mood you want to create. Soft lighting and gentle music can set a relaxed atmosphere, while upbeat tunes and lively decor can energize the evening. Offer guests the chance to get hands-on experience with interactive mocktail stations and experiment with their own seasonal twists. With these ideas in mind, you're well-equipped to embrace the seasons with mocktails that taste as good as they look.

Pairing Mocktails with Food: A Culinary Guide

Pairing drinks with food is a bit like matchmaking. It's finding the harmony where flavors sing together like a well-rehearsed choir. When it comes to mocktails, the principles are no different from traditional pairings. You want to balance flavors, allowing the drink to complement or contrast with the dish, enhancing the overall dining experience. Think about how a sweet, refreshing mocktail might soften the heat of a spicy dish or how a tangy, citrusy beverage can cut through the richness of a creamy sauce. It's all about finding that balance—like wearing a chunky knit sweater with a sleek pair of jeans.

Take the **Virgin Sangria**, for instance. Its rich, fruity notes pair beautifully with Spanish tapas. The Sangria's sweetness and fruitiness complement the salty, savory flavors of the dishes, creating a delightful dance on the palate. Or consider the **Cucumber Lime Cooler** paired with sushi. The cool, crisp mocktail mirrors the freshness of the sushi, while the lime adds a citrusy zing that brightens each bite. And then there's the **Ginger Lemonade**, a mocktail that pairs wonderfully with BBQ dishes. The ginger provides a spicy kick, while the lemonade offers a refreshing contrast to BBQ's hearty, smoky flavors, making each bite feel lighter and more vibrant.

Mocktails do more than accompany a meal—they elevate it. A well-paired mocktail can enhance the flavor profiles of a dish, acting as a palate cleanser between courses. This refreshes the taste buds, preparing them for the next culinary adventure. It's like hitting the reset button, ensuring each bite feels as exciting as the first. When crafting a mocktail and food menu, consider the flavors and textures of both the drinks and the dishes. Plan a multi-course meal where each mocktail complements or contrasts with the food, creating a cohesive dining experience. Don't forget to consider dietary restrictions and preferences, ensuring something for everyone. This thoughtful approach not only impresses your guests but also transforms a simple meal into a memorable occasion.

DIY MOCKTAIL MIXERS AND GARNISHES

Imagine you're in your kitchen, surrounded by the enticing aroma of fresh ingredients, ready to concoct your own mocktail mixers and garnishes. Crafting these elements at home allows you to tailor flavors precisely to your palate and also ensures you know exactly what's going into your drink. No more mystery ingredients or preservatives here. With DIY mixers, you can experiment with flavors, creating a unique blend that makes your mocktail truly your own. Plus, there's something immensely satisfying about sipping on a drink that you've crafted from scratch.

Start with simple recipes like homemade grenadine, which transforms pomegranate juice and sugar into a sweet syrup that adds a vibrant red hue to any drink. Or try your hand at a lavender simple syrup, where sugar, water, and dried lavender blossoms come together to create a floral concoction that can elevate any mocktail. Fresh fruit purees are another fantastic addition. Blend seasonal fruits like strawberries or peaches and strain them to make a smooth, flavorful base. These mixers serve as the foundation, offering endless possibilities for creativity with every pour.

Now, let's talk garnishes. Elevate your mocktails with unique and visually stunning garnishes to make your drinks the star of any gathering. Edible flowers, like violets or nasturtiums, add a splash of color and a hint of floral flavor. Dehydrated fruit slices, whether lemon, lime, or orange, look chic and infuse a subtle citrus note as they rehydrate. Herb sprigs and zest ribbons, such as rosemary or lemon peel, can add layers of aroma and flavor, turning a simple drink into a multisensory experience.

Properly storing your homemade mixers and garnishes is crucial to maintaining freshness and flavor. Store syrups in the refrigerator in an airtight container, where they'll keep for up to a month. Dehydrated fruits and herbs should be kept in a cool, dark place to preserve their vibrant colors and flavors. And don't let leftovers go to waste—use them creatively! Stir leftover lavender syrup into a cup of tea for a soothing afternoon break, or sprinkle dehydrated fruit over your morning cereal. With these tips in mind, your mocktail-making skills will reach new heights, delighting your taste buds and guests' eyes with every sip.

BEYOND MOCKTAILS: EXPLORING OTHER NON-ALCOHOLIC BEVERAGES

Let's wander off the beaten path of mocktails and explore a world brimming with refreshing non-alcoholic beverages. Infused waters are like nature's spa day in a glass, offering hydration with a twist. Combine slices of cucumber and fresh mint leaves in a water pitcher, and let the flavors meld in the fridge for a few hours. The result is a crisp, refreshing drink that quenches your thirst and feels like a mini-vacation for your palate. For those who fancy a warm, calming sip, herbal teas and tisanes are a delightful choice. Picture a steaming cup of Chamomile Lavender Tea, made by steeping chamomile flowers and lavender buds in hot water. This soothing concoction is perfect for winding down after a long day, offering a gentle embrace of tranquility.

Smoothies and shakes, on the other hand, are the colorful, nutrient-packed powerhouses of the beverage world. Imagine a **Green Detox Smoothie**, a verdant blend of spinach, kale, banana, and a splash of almond milk. This vibrant drink is a feast for the eyes and a nutritional powerhouse, rich in vitamins and minerals that support overall wellness. These alternative beverages do more than taste good—they provide essential hydration and detoxification, helping to flush out toxins and replenish your body's needs. They are your allies in maintaining balance and vitality, supporting your physical and mental well-being.

Getting creative with these drinks is a breeze. Play around with different herbs, fruits, and flavor intensities to craft a beverage that suits your taste buds. Try mixing basil with strawberries for a refreshing twist on infused water, or add a pinch of turmeric to your smoothie for an anti-inflammatory boost. Adjust sweetness levels to your preference, perhaps with a hint of honey or a splash of agave. The beauty of these non-alcoholic options is their versatility and adaptability, allowing you to tailor each sip to your liking.

CREATING YOUR SIGNATURE MOCKTAIL

Creating your signature mocktail is like painting a masterpiece on a blank canvas. It starts with choosing a base flavor profile that speaks to your taste buds. Maybe you're drawn to the refreshing zest of citrus or the soothing aroma of herbs. Once you've settled on a base, let the experimentation begin! Mix and match different ingredients like a mad scientist, testing out unique combinations that might surprise you.

Strawberry and basil? Why not? Cucumber and ginger? Go for it! The key is to play and have fun, letting your inner mixologist lead the way.

Achieving that perfect balance of flavors and textures is akin to conducting a symphony. You want your creation to hit the right notes of sweetness and acidity, perhaps with a hint of bitterness to keep things interesting. Adjust the sweetness by adding or reducing syrups, and play with acidity using citrus juices. Don't forget texture—consider adding a frothy top with a splash of egg white or a fizzy finish with a dash of soda. It's all about creating a drink that tastes good and feels good on the palate, offering a complete sensory experience.

Once you've concocted your masterpiece, it's time to give it a name that captures its essence. Think about personal inspirations or themes that might guide you. It may remind you of a favorite vacation spot or a cherished memory. Incorporate puns or wordplay for a touch of humor—something like "Mint to Be" or "Berry Happy." The name should be as unique as the drink itself, leaving an impression that sticks long after the last sip.

Presenting your signature mocktail is an opportunity to showcase your creativity. Use stylish glassware that complements the drink's color and vibe. Add garnishes that pop, like a twist of lemon peel or a sprig of rosemary, to elevate the presentation. Share your creation with friends and family by hosting a tasting party or sharing the recipe. Encourage them to try making it themselves, turning your signature mocktail into a shared experience that brings people together.

9

LONG-TERM SUCCESS AND LIFESTYLE CHANGES

I magine you've just finished a marathon. Your legs are jelly, but your spirit is soaring. That's Dry January for you—a month-long marathon of willpower and self-discovery. Now that you've reached the finish line, it's time to take a deep breath and reflect on this monumental achievement. Grab a comfy seat, maybe a cup of tea, and let's dive into the wealth of insights you've gathered. This isn't just about patting yourself on the back (though you should definitely do that); it's about understanding the journey you took and the lessons it brought you.

REFLECTING ON YOUR DRY JANUARY JOURNEY

Reflecting on your experiences is like revisiting a favorite novel, finding new layers and depths you didn't notice before. Think about the key moments that stood out, both the highs and the lows. What surprised you? What made you laugh, cry, or want to throw in the towel? Journaling these reflections can illuminate patterns and triggers, helping to prepare for future challenges. Consider prompts like, "What was my biggest challenge, and how did I overcome it?" or "What was my proudest moment?" These questions can guide you in exploring personal growth, revealing strengths you didn't know you had. Perhaps you discovered a knack for mocktail mixology or found comfort in an evening walk.

Dry January is a masterclass in self-awareness. Recognizing your triggers is like finding the "off" switch on a noisy appliance—life becomes a little quieter and more manageable. Did you find that stress made you reach for a glass, or was it the allure of a social gathering? Understanding these triggers allows you to devise coping strategies, like replacing a drink with a healthier habit. This month, you probably revealed some of your personal strengths. Maybe you have an iron willpower or a newfound love for early mornings. But it's also okay to acknowledge weaknesses, as they are stepping stones to growth. Perhaps you realized that a lack of planning led to temptation, a lesson for future endeavors.

Successes, both big and small, deserve a spotlight. Celebrate those milestones like a personal holiday. Whether it's surviving a party without a drink or saving enough money for a treat, these victories are yours to cherish. Plan a meaningful reward—maybe a fancy dinner or a day out doing something you love. Share your triumphs with friends and family, inviting them to join the celebration. Not only does this reinforce your achievements, but it also strengthens your support network, creating a circle of encouragement and inspiration.

Of course, every journey comes with its fair share of bumps and detours. It is important to reflect honestly on the challenges faced during Dry January. What were the most challenging moments? How did you navigate them? Identifying areas for improvement is like refining a recipe—each tweak brings you closer to perfection. Use these insights to develop strategies for future obstacles. If stress was a trigger, consider incorporating relaxation techniques. If social settings were difficult, explore new ways to socialize without alcohol.

Journaling Prompts for Reflection

- What was the biggest challenge you faced, and how did you overcome it?
- Describe a moment you felt proud of yourself during Dry January.
- How did you cope with cravings or social pressure?
- What new habits or routines did you enjoy?
- How will you apply the lessons learned to future challenges?

Reflecting on Dry January isn't just about looking back; it's about preparing for the future. These insights are your toolkit, ready to support you in maintaining your progress and guiding you in future alcohol-free endeavors.

TURNING DRY JANUARY INTO A LONG-TERM COMMITMENT

As you roll off the Dry January train, you might find yourself basking in the glow of accomplishment, wondering, "What's next?" The truth is, the end of January doesn't have to mean the end of your alcohol-free days. There are ways to extend the momentum and keep the good vibes rolling. Consider participating in future sobriety challenges like Sober October or No-Drinks November. These events provide perfect opportunities to revisit your goals and continue reaping the benefits of an alcohol-free lifestyle. Setting extended sobriety goals is like drawing up a game plan for your personal championship—clear, intentional, and full of promise. Create a support plan to ensure you're not riding solo. Enlist your friends, family, or even your dog for emotional backing. Think of it as building a team of cheerleaders who won't judge you for drinking kombucha instead of craft beer.

Sustaining an alcohol-free lifestyle goes beyond just saying no to drinks at happy hour. It's about embracing the ongoing health improvements that come with it. Remember the surprising boost of energy you felt? The clearer skin and the weight loss weren't figments of your imagination. They're the tangible perks of giving your body a break from booze, and they keep on giving. Your liver thanks you, your brain thanks you, and even your wallet gives a silent nod of approval. Those financial savings you pocketed in January? They multiply when you continue this lifestyle. The financial freedom is a sweet bonus, whether extra cash for a dream vacation or just padding your savings account. Life without alcohol is like finding a secret level in a game where the rewards keep coming.

Now, staying the course isn't always easy without a safety net. Luckily, plenty of support systems are available. Online communities and forums are buzzing with folks just like you, swapping stories, tips, and even the occasional virtual high-five. Dive into spaces like Reddit's r/stopdrinking or dedicated Facebook groups to find camaraderie and encouragement. These communities are vibrant, judgment-free zones where you can engage with others who share your goals. On a more local level, many areas offer support groups and networks designed to help people maintain sobriety. Whether a weekly meeting at a community center or a casual gathering at a coffee shop, these groups provide a sense of belonging and a platform to share your experiences.

Taking the leap into long-term sobriety can be daunting, but armed with the right strategies, it's entirely doable. Set clear intentions and goals, much like planning a road trip. Know your destination, pack your bags, and prepare for detours. Having a map makes the journey smoother, and you're more likely to arrive at your destination with a smile on your face. Remember, this isn't about perfection. It's about progress and finding what works best for you. Whether you choose to participate in another month-long challenge or adopt a more flexible approach, the key is to remain open to the ongoing benefits. So, go ahead and embrace the positive changes you've started. Take pride in your achievements and keep the momentum going. After all, who doesn't want a life filled with clarity, health, and a little extra cash?

SETTING NEW GOALS FOR CONTINUED SUCCESS

Setting new goals is like plotting the coordinates for the adventure ahead. It's what keeps the momentum going, ensuring that progress doesn't stall like a car out of gas. The role of goal-setting in maintaining progress cannot be overstated. Personal goals are your North Star, guiding you towards a fulfilling life aligned with your values. Maybe it's about climbing the corporate ladder, or perhaps it's about nurturing your creative side. Professional aspirations can fuel your journey toward career advancement and skill-building, opening doors you didn't even know were there. Health and wellness objectives, on the other hand, are the bedrock of a thriving life. Whether it's running that 5k you've always talked about or mastering the art of meditation, these goals anchor your well-being in a sea of possibilities.

But let's talk strategy. A framework for goal-setting is like a trusty map in unfamiliar territory. Enter the SMART goals framework: Specific, Measurable, Achievable, Relevant, and Time-bound—these pillars transform nebulous dreams into tangible realities. Specific goals are unambiguous, like "I will run three times a week," instead of "I'll exercise more." Measurable goals let you track progress to know when you've hit the mark. Achievable goals are within reach, challenging yet feasible, ensuring you're not setting yourself up for disappointment. Relevant goals align with your broader life objectives, making sure every step is meaningful. Time-bound goals come with a deadline, creating a sense of urgency that propels you forward.

Now, why not spice things up? Diversifying your goals adds richness and variety to your life. Think of it as a buffet of opportunities—career goals, personal development, hobbies, and more. Maybe you've always wanted to learn a new language or take up sculpting. Perhaps you're eager to dive into a new field of study or expand your professional network. The beauty of diversified goals is that they cater to all aspects of your life, creating a balanced tapestry of experiences.

In the wise words of Ralph Waldo Emerson, "The only person you are destined to become is the person you decide to be." Embrace the power of goal-setting as you continue this path of self-discovery and growth. Choose goals that resonate with your heart's desires and align with your vision for the future. Whether it's personal, professional, or somewhere in between, your goals are the stepping stones to a life of purpose and possibility.

MAINTAINING HEALTHY HABITS YEAR-ROUND

Imagine your health habits as a trusty old bicycle. It takes a little effort to keep it moving, but once you're cruising, it feels like you're flying. Consistent healthy habits are the spokes in the wheel of long-term success. They keep you steady and prevent you from wobbling back into old patterns. Building a sustainable lifestyle is like creating a playlist of your favorite songs—each habit adds rhythm and joy to your life. It's about making choices that align with your values and goals, creating an authentic and fulfilling life. When you maintain these habits, you're avoiding relapse and crafting a life supporting your deepest aspirations.

Physical health is your foundation, the bedrock upon which everything else is built. Regular exercise routines are like brushing your teeth—they're non-negotiable for a healthy life. Find activities that you love, whether it's dancing like nobody's watching or going for a brisk walk in the park. Exercise keeps your body strong and your mind sharp. Balanced and nutritious meal planning is the fuel for this well-oiled machine. Think of your body as a gourmet kitchen—stock it with whole grains, lean proteins, and colorful veggies, and you'll whip up meals that nourish your body and soul. Practical tips like prepping meals in advance or swapping out sugary snacks for fruits can make all the difference.

Mental and emotional well-being are the secret sauce to a happy life. Mindfulness and relaxation techniques are like mini-vacations for your mind. Take a few minutes each day to breathe deeply, meditate, or simply enjoy a quiet moment of reflection. Regular self-care practices are your safety net. It might be a hot bath, a good book, or a stroll in nature—whatever soothes your spirit and recharges your batteries. Prioritizing these moments is essential for maintaining equilibrium in a busy world. A healthy mind is a fertile ground for creativity, problem-solving, and joy.

It's about making choices that align with your true self and creating a rich and rewarding life. So, hop on that bicycle and pedal towards a life filled with joy, health, and vitality.

INSPIRING OTHERS WITH YOUR STORY

Have you ever considered how powerful your story could be? Sharing your journey through Dry January or any other alcohol-free adventure isn't just about airing your laundry or bragging about your achievements. It's about connecting with others and building a sense of community. Think of it like a ripple effect. You toss a pebble into the pond by sharing your experiences, and suddenly, those ripples are reaching people you never imagined. Your story can be the nudge someone else needs to embark on their own path to sobriety. When you speak about your challenges and victories, you offer a relatable narrative that others can latch onto. People see themselves in your triumphs and struggles, and that connection can be profoundly motivating. Plus, there's something invigorating about knowing you're not just walking this path alone. You're part of something bigger that collectively encourages support and inspires change.

So, how do you go about sharing your story effectively? First off, let's talk platforms. Writing blog posts or social media updates can be a great start. Not only do these formats allow for a wide reach, but they also encourage interaction. You might find that others are eager to share their own experiences in response, creating a dialogue that benefits everyone involved. Consider speaking at local events or support groups if you're feeling courageous. Your voice can resonate in ways you might not expect, and face-to-face interaction can be incredibly powerful. When you share, be authentic. People appreciate honesty and vulnerability. It's not about putting on a brave face but being genuine and sharing the ups and downs. Remember, authenticity breeds connection.

As you continue on your path, consider stepping into a mentoring role. Becoming a sobriety mentor or coach can be incredibly rewarding for you and those you support. Offer your insights to friends or family who may be contemplating sobriety. Sometimes, all it takes is a gentle nudge from someone who's been there. By sharing your journey, you reinforce your commitment and inspire and hope for others. It's about paying it forward, offering guidance and encouragement to those who might feel lost or unsure. You'll find that supporting others is a two-way street. Not only do you help them grow, but you'll also discover new insights about yourself, deepening your understanding and commitment to a sober lifestyle. Your story is a powerful tool—wield it with empathy and purpose.

10

MOCKTAIL RECIPE GUIDE

SIMPLE GO-TO COCKTAILS

Apple Cinnamon Refresher

- Ingredients: 6 oz apple juice, pinch of cinnamon
- Instructions: Add cinnamon to apple juice, serve over ice.

Apple Ginger Fizz

- Ingredients: 6 oz apple juice, 4 oz ginger ale, 1 cinnamon stick
- Instructions: Mix apple juice and ginger ale, garnish with a cinnamon stick.

Apple Mint Refresher

- Ingredients: 6 oz apple juice, 6 mint leaves, 4 oz sparkling water
- Instructions: Mix apple juice with mint and sparkling water.

Berry Lemonade

- Ingredients: ½ cup mixed berries, 8 oz lemonade
- Instructions: Blend berries with lemonade. Serve over ice.

Blackberry Lime Fizz

- Ingredients: ½ cup blackberries, juice of 1 lime, 8 oz soda water
- Instructions: Muddle blackberries with lime juice, add soda water.

Blueberry Mint Fizz

- Ingredients: ½ cup blueberries, 6 mint leaves, 8 oz soda water
- Instructions: Muddle blueberries and mint, pour over ice, and top with soda water.

Blood Orange Fizz

- Ingredients: 4 oz blood orange juice, 4 oz soda water
- Instructions: Mix blood orange juice with soda water over ice.

Cherry Berry Fizz

- Ingredients: 4 oz cherry juice, ½ cup mixed berries, 6 oz soda water
- Instructions: Combine cherry juice with berries and soda water.

Cherry Limeade

- Ingredients: 4 oz cherry juice, juice of 1 lime, 4 oz soda water
- Instructions: Mix cherry juice and lime juice over ice, add soda water.

Citrus Basil Smash

- Ingredients: 6 basil leaves, 3 oz orange juice, 1 oz lemon juice
- Instructions: Muddle basil, add orange and lemon juice. Pour over ice and stir.

Cranberry Lime Sparkler

- Ingredients: 4 oz cranberry juice, juice of 1 lime, 4 oz sparkling water
- Instructions: Mix cranberry and lime juice, top with sparkling water.

Cranberry Spritzer

- Ingredients: 6 oz cranberry juice, 4 oz sparkling water, 1 lime wedge
- Instructions: Mix cranberry juice and sparkling water. Serve over ice with a lime wedge.

Cucumber Cooler

- Ingredients: ½ cucumber (sliced), 1 oz lemon juice, 8 oz soda water
- Instructions: Muddle cucumber, add lemon juice and ice. Top with soda water and stir.

Cucumber Ginger Cooler

- Ingredients: ½ cucumber, 6 oz ginger ale
- Instructions: Muddle cucumber, top with ginger ale.

Cucumber Mint Sparkler

- Ingredients: ½ cucumber, 6 mint leaves, 8 oz sparkling water
- Instructions: Muddle cucumber and mint, top with sparkling water.

Coconut Lime Refresher

- Ingredients: 6 oz coconut water, juice of 1 lime, 6 mint leaves
- Instructions: Combine coconut water and lime juice. Garnish with mint.

Ginger Lime Tonic

- Ingredients: 8 oz ginger ale, juice of 1 lime
- Instructions: Combine ginger ale and lime juice over ice. Garnish with lime.

Grapefruit Basil Sparkler

- Ingredients: 4 oz grapefruit juice, 6 basil leaves, 6 oz soda water
- Instructions: Muddle basil, add grapefruit juice and soda water.

Honey Ginger Lemonade

- Ingredients: 2 oz lemon juice, 1 tbsp honey, 6 oz ginger ale
- Instructions: Mix lemon juice and honey, top with ginger ale.

Lavender Lemonade

- Ingredients: 1 tbsp lavender syrup, 8 oz lemonade
- Instructions: Mix lavender syrup and lemonade over ice.

Lemon Basil Sparkler

- Ingredients: 5 basil leaves, 2 oz lemon juice, 6 oz sparkling water
- Instructions: Muddle basil and lemon juice, add sparkling water.

Lemon Mint Cooler

- Ingredients: 2 oz lemon juice, 6 mint leaves, 8 oz soda water
- Instructions: Muddle mint and lemon juice, add soda water.

Mango Lemonade

- Ingredients: 3 oz mango puree, 6 oz lemonade
- Instructions: Mix mango puree and lemonade over ice.

Mint Julep Mocktail

- Ingredients: 6 mint leaves, 1 tsp sugar, 6 oz soda water
- Instructions: Muddle mint and sugar, add ice and soda water.

Minty Pomegranate Cooler

- Ingredients: 6 oz pomegranate juice, 8 mint leaves, 4 oz soda water
- Instructions: Muddle mint with pomegranate juice. Add soda water and serve over ice.

Orange Cranberry Cooler

- Ingredients: 4 oz orange juice, 4 oz cranberry juice
- Instructions: Combine juices, serve over ice.

Orange Creamsicle Mocktail

- Ingredients: 4 oz orange juice, 4 oz vanilla almond milk
- Instructions: Mix orange juice with vanilla almond milk. Serve over ice.

Passion Fruit Cooler

- Ingredients: 4 oz passion fruit juice, 4 oz soda water
- Instructions: Mix passion fruit juice with soda water over ice.

Peach Iced Tea

- Ingredients: 2 oz peach puree, 8 oz iced tea
- Instructions: Mix peach puree with iced tea over ice.

Pineapple Ginger Beer Mocktail

- Ingredients: 4 oz pineapple juice, 4 oz ginger beer, juice of 1 lime
- Instructions: Pour pineapple juice and ginger beer over ice. Garnish with a lime wedge.

Pomegranate Lime Sparkler

- Ingredients: 6 oz pomegranate juice, juice of 1 lime, 4 oz sparkling water
- Instructions: Mix pomegranate juice and lime, add sparkling water.

Raspberry Lemon Fizz

- Ingredients: ½ cup raspberries, 1 oz lemon juice, 6 oz sparkling water
- Instructions: Muddle raspberries with lemon juice, add sparkling water.

Rosewater Lemonade

- Ingredients: 1 tsp rosewater, 8 oz lemonade
- Instructions: Mix rosewater with lemonade.

Rosemary Grapefruit Fizz

- Ingredients: 6 oz grapefruit juice, 4 oz soda water, 1 rosemary sprig
- Instructions: Pour grapefruit juice and soda water over ice. Garnish with rosemary.

Sparkling Apple Lemonade

- Ingredients: 4 oz apple juice, 4 oz lemonade, 4 oz sparkling water
- Instructions: Mix apple juice, lemonade, and sparkling water.

Sparkling Hibiscus Mocktail

- Ingredients: 4 oz brewed hibiscus tea, 4 oz sparkling water
- Instructions: Brew hibiscus tea, cool, and mix with sparkling water.

Spiced Apple Cider

- Ingredients: 8 oz apple cider, 1 cinnamon stick, pinch of nutmeg
- Instructions: Heat apple cider with cinnamon and nutmeg.

Spiced Citrus Punch

- Ingredients: 4 oz orange juice, 2 oz lemon juice, pinch of cinnamon
- Instructions: Combine juices, add a dash of cinnamon.

Strawberry Basil Lemonade

- Ingredients: ½ cup strawberries, 5 basil leaves, 6 oz lemonade
- Instructions: Muddle strawberries and basil, add lemonade over ice.

Strawberry Lemonade

- Ingredients: ½ cup strawberries, 2 oz lemon juice, 6 oz sparkling water
- Instructions: Blend strawberries and lemon juice. Pour over ice and top with sparkling water.

Tropical Punch

- Ingredients: 4 oz pineapple juice, 2 oz orange juice, 2 oz cranberry juice
- Instructions: Mix all juices and serve over ice.

Virgin Bellini

- Ingredients: 2 oz peach puree, 6 oz sparkling water
- Instructions: Mix peach puree with sparkling water. Serve chilled.

Virgin Mimosa

- Ingredients: 4 oz orange juice, 4 oz sparkling water
- Instructions: Combine orange juice and sparkling water over ice.

Virgin Mojito

- Ingredients: 10 mint leaves, 1 oz lime juice, 1 tsp sugar, 8 oz soda water
- Instructions: Muddle mint, sugar, and lime in a glass, add ice, and top with soda water. Stir well.

Virgin Moscow Mule

- Ingredients: 8 oz ginger beer, juice of 1 lime
- Instructions: Combine ginger beer and lime juice over ice.

Virgin Piña Colada

- Ingredients: 6 oz coconut milk, 6 oz pineapple juice
- Instructions: Blend coconut milk and pineapple juice. Serve over ice.

Virgin Sangria

- Ingredients: 4 oz orange juice, 4 oz apple juice, ½ cup mixed berries
- Instructions: Mix juices, add berries, serve chilled.

Virgin Sunset

- Ingredients: 6 oz orange juice, 1 oz grenadine
- Instructions: Pour orange juice, add grenadine to create a sunset effect.

Virgin Strawberry Daiquiri

- Ingredients: ½ cup strawberries, juice of 1 lime
- Instructions: Blend strawberries with lime juice.

MORE COMPLEX MOCKTAILS

Berry Basil Sparkling Mocktail

This drink has complex berry, citrus, and herbal notes, layered with a tangy basil foam on top for a unique and elevated look.

Ingredients:

- 1 oz fresh blackberry puree
- 1 oz fresh raspberry puree
- ½ oz lemon juice
- 1 oz basil syrup (recipe below)
- 3 oz sparkling water
- 1 fresh basil leaf and berries for garnish

For the Basil Syrup:

- ½ cup water
- ½ cup sugar
- 10 fresh basil leaves

For the Basil Foam:

- 1 oz basil syrup
- 1 oz lemon juice
- 2 oz aquafaba (liquid from canned chickpeas) or 1 egg white

Instructions:

- Make the Basil Syrup: Combine water and sugar in a saucepan, bring to a simmer, and add basil leaves. Steep for 10 minutes, then strain and let cool.
- Prepare the Foam: In a shaker, combine basil syrup, lemon juice, and aquafaba (or egg white). Shake vigorously until a thick foam forms.

- Mix the Mocktail: In another shaker, combine the blackberry puree, raspberry puree, lemon juice, and 1 oz basil syrup with ice. Shake and strain into a glass with ice.
- Layer and Garnish: Slowly top with sparkling water, then gently spoon the basil foam on top.
- Garnish: Add a basil leaf and a few fresh berries for a dramatic presentation.

Berry Herb Elixir

This mocktail layers berry, citrus, and herbal notes for a refreshing and sophisticated drink, garnished with a fruit skewer and fragrant herbs.

Ingredients:

- ½ cup mixed berries (such as blueberries, blackberries, raspberries)
- 1 tbsp honey or agave syrup
- 2 oz fresh lemon juice
- 3 oz hibiscus tea (brewed and cooled)
- 2 oz sparkling water
- 2–3 fresh thyme sprigs
- 2–3 fresh mint leaves
- Ice
- Garnish: Mixed berry skewer and fresh thyme or mint sprig

Instructions:

- In a shaker, muddle the berries with honey and lemon juice until well combined.
- Clap the thyme sprigs and mint leaves between your hands to release their aroma, then add them to the shaker.
- Add the hibiscus tea and ice, then shake vigorously for 20–30 seconds.
- Strain into a glass with fresh ice and top with sparkling water.
- Garnish with a berry skewer and a sprig of thyme or mint.

Herbal Blackberry Sage Smash

This earthy, berry-infused mocktail combines blackberries, sage, and lemon with a hint of honey.

Ingredients:

- ½ cup fresh blackberries
- 4–6 fresh sage leaves
- ½ oz honey syrup (equal parts honey and warm water)
- ½ oz lemon juice
- 2 oz cranberry juice
- 4 oz soda water
- Crushed ice
- Garnish: Blackberry and sage for garnish

Instructions:

- In a shaker, muddle blackberries, sage leaves, honey syrup, and lemon juice until the mixture is well combined.
- Add cranberry juice and fill the shaker halfway with ice. Shake vigorously.
- Strain the mixture into a glass filled with crushed ice.
- Top with soda water and gently stir.
- Garnish with a blackberry and a sage leaf for a visually appealing finish.

Pineapple Sage Elixir

This layered mocktail combines herbal and tropical flavors with a striking presentation.

Ingredients:

- 2 oz fresh pineapple juice
- 1 oz lime juice
- 1 oz sage syrup (recipe below)
- 2 oz cold-brewed green tea

- 2 oz sparkling water
- Pineapple slice and fresh sage leaves for garnish

For the Sage Syrup:

- ½ cup water
- ½ cup sugar
- 5 fresh sage leaves

Instructions:

- Make the Sage Syrup: In a small saucepan, bring water and sugar to a boil, then add sage leaves. Simmer for 5 minutes, then let cool. Remove the sage leaves and strain.
- In a shaker, combine the pineapple juice, lime juice, and 1 oz of sage syrup. Add ice and shake well.
- Strain into a tall glass filled with ice, then slowly pour the green tea over a spoon to create a layered effect.
- Top with sparkling water and garnish with a pineapple slice and a few sage leaves.

Spiced Hibiscus Berry Sparkler

This refreshing mocktail combines spiced hibiscus tea, mixed berry syrup, and a fizzy finish.

Ingredients:

- 4 oz brewed hibiscus tea (cooled)
- 1 oz homemade berry syrup (see recipe below)
- 1 oz fresh lime juice
- 1-2 oz ginger beer or sparkling water
- Fresh mint leaves
- Fresh berries (for garnish)

Berry Syrup Recipe:

- ½ cup mixed berries (blueberries, raspberries, or blackberries)
- ¼ cup water
- 1 tbsp honey or sugar

Instructions for Berry Syrup:

- Combine berries, water, and honey (or sugar) in a small saucepan. Simmer over low heat for 5-7 minutes, until berries break down and the mixture thickens.
- Strain the syrup through a fine mesh sieve, pressing down to extract all liquid. Let cool.

Mocktail Instructions:

- In a shaker, combine the hibiscus tea, berry syrup, and lime juice. Shake with ice to chill and mix.
- Pour into a glass over ice, and top with ginger beer or sparkling water for a touch of fizz.
- Garnish with fresh mint leaves and a few berries for a burst of color and freshness.

Spiced Orange Ginger Fizz

This zesty, spiced mocktail combines fresh orange juice, ginger, cinnamon, and a splash of sparkling water.

Ingredients:

- 1 orange, juiced (about 3 oz)
- ½ oz ginger syrup (or 1 inch fresh ginger, sliced and muddled)
- ¼ tsp ground cinnamon or a cinnamon stick
- ½ oz lemon juice
- ½ oz honey syrup
- 2 oz soda water or tonic water
- Orange slice and cinnamon stick for garnish

- Crushed ice

Instructions:

- In a shaker, combine orange juice, ginger syrup, cinnamon, lemon juice, and honey syrup. Shake well with ice to chill.
- Strain into a glass filled with crushed ice.
- Top with soda water or tonic water and stir gently to mix.
- Garnish with an orange slice and a cinnamon stick for extra spice and aroma.

Tropical Layered Sunset

This mocktail has beautiful color layers and a vibrant tropical taste.

Ingredients:

- 3 oz pineapple juice
- 3 oz mango juice
- 1 oz grenadine
- 1 oz coconut milk
- 1 oz orange juice
- Ice cubes
- Fresh pineapple or a cherry for garnish

Instructions:

- Bottom Layer: Pour grenadine into the bottom of a tall glass to create the rich, sunset color at the base.
- Middle Layer: In a shaker, combine the pineapple juice and mango juice with ice. Carefully pour this mixture over the back of a spoon into the glass, layering it over the grenadine. This should create a clear layer above the grenadine.
- Top Layer: Combine the coconut milk and orange juice in a shaker with ice, shake gently. Using the back of a spoon, layer this mix over the pineapple-mango layer to add a creamy, tropical top.

- Garnish: Add a pineapple slice or a cherry. The layered effect mimics a tropical sunset, and the flavors are just as vibrant!

Tropical Spice Fusion

A multi-layered drink that combines tropical fruits, spices, and fresh herbs for a refreshing, warming mocktail.

Ingredients:

- 4 oz pineapple juice
- 2 oz coconut water
- 1 oz fresh orange juice
- 1 oz fresh lime juice
- 1 tbsp ginger syrup (recipe below)
- ¼ tsp cinnamon
- ½ tsp vanilla extract
- 2–3 basil leaves
- 2–3 thin cucumber slices
- Ice
- Optional Garnish: Pineapple slice, basil sprig, or cinnamon stick

Instructions:

- In a shaker, add pineapple juice, coconut water, orange juice, lime juice, ginger syrup, cinnamon, and vanilla.
- Clap the basil leaves between your hands to release their aroma and add them to the shaker along with the cucumber slices.
- Add ice and shake vigorously for 20–30 seconds.
- Strain the mixture into a tall glass over fresh ice.
- Garnish with a pineapple slice, basil sprig, or a cinnamon stick for an added aromatic touch.

Ginger Syrup Recipe:

- In a small saucepan, combine 1 cup sugar, 1 cup water, and a 2-inch piece of fresh ginger (sliced).
- Bring to a simmer, stirring until the sugar dissolves, then let it simmer for 5 minutes.
- Remove from heat, let cool, and strain out the ginger pieces.

YOUR SUPPORT IS EXTREMELY IMPORTANT!

Now that you have the insights and tools to embrace a healthier, alcohol-free lifestyle, it's time to share your newfound knowledge and guide others to discover the same transformative benefits.

By leaving your honest opinion of this book on Amazon, you'll help others looking to manage their alcohol consumption, enhance their well-being, and achieve their personal goals for Dry January, Sober October, or any month you choose to abstain from alcohol. Your review can inspire and support individuals on their journey toward better health and mental clarity.

Promoting a mindful approach to alcohol consumption thrives when we share our experiences—you play a vital role in helping others continue this important work. Your voice matters, and your review can lead others to follow.

It's simple to leave a review on Amazon: Visit the book's Amazon **'Write a customer review'** page by simply scanning the link below.

Your support is extremely important to us. Great things can happen from a small gesture!

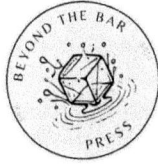
BEYOND THE BAR PRESS

CONCLUSION

And here we are at the finish line—what an incredible journey! Together, we've delved into the vibrant world of mocktails, discovered effective ways to reduce alcohol consumption, and embraced a healthier, clearer, and more fulfilling lifestyle—for both your spirit and your wallet. "Mocktails over Cocktails" was designed to equip you with the tools and inspiration to navigate challenges like Dry January and Sober October with grace and confidence. We hope you feel empowered and ready to tackle your next adventure.

Remember the valuable insights you uncovered along the way? The sense of accomplishment that comes from waking up without a hangover? The excitement of exploring new hobbies and passions? And the simple pleasure of enjoying a perfectly crafted mocktail—proof that social gatherings can be enjoyable without the next-day regrets.

As we wrap up, here's a heartfelt message from all of us at Beyond the Bar Press. Our mission has always been to support you in navigating the sometimes challenging path of sobriety. It has been a pleasure to accompany you on this journey. Seeing individuals embrace change and discover new facets of their lives drives us every day. Thank you for allowing us to be a part of your story.

To everyone who has successfully completed Dry January or any other sober challenge—give yourself a well-deserved high five! You've persevered and thrived, gaining invaluable insights and personal growth along the way. Whether you've developed a passion for mocktail mixology or found joy in waking up refreshed on weekends, each step forward is a victory. Be proud of your accomplishments. Redefining your relationship with alcohol is no small feat, and every moment of progress deserves celebration.

But remember, this isn't the end—it's the beginning of a new chapter. Consider setting new goals to maintain your momentum. Perhaps incorporate regular alcohol-free days into your routine or embark on another sober challenge. These small adjustments can help sustain your newfound clarity and energy.

And don't keep your success to yourself! Share your journey with your community—whether through social media, local support groups, or conversations with friends. Your story could inspire someone else to start their own path. Connecting with others who share similar goals can also provide a supportive network that makes the journey even more rewarding.

As you move forward, carry with you the lessons you've learned. Embrace the positive changes and the healthier, happier version of yourself that has emerged. You are part of a growing community of individuals choosing mindful living and sobriety, and that is something to be proud of.

So here's to you—your resilience, your determination, and your bright future. May your days be filled with clarity, your nights with peace, and your life with the joys of mindful living. Cheers to a healthier, happier you!

REFERENCES

5 Women Share The Benefits of Dry January https://www.womenshealthmag.com/health/a19932399/dry-january-experiences/

6 Alcohol-Free Ways to Unwind at the End of a Long Day https://www.everydayhealth.com/self-care/alcohol-free-ways-to-unwind-at-the-end-of-a-long-day/

7 Foods That Can Help Stop Alcohol Cravings https://compassionbehavioralhealth.com/7-foods-that-can-help-stop-alcohol-cravings/

8 Ways to Turn Down Alcohol if You Aren't Drinking https://www.healthline.com/health/alcohol/say-no-to-alcohol

9 Health Benefits of Not Drinking Alcohol Backed By Science https://www.drinksurely.com/a/blog/benefits-of-not-drinking-alcohol?srsltid=AfmBOorHCiVtTBJQGK5Vgn-PkD2anYNwRZIU0w_bXX_IaMC9D1HPCC846

21 Mindfulness Exercises & Activities For Adults (+ PDF) https://positivepsychology.com/mindfulness-exercises-techniques-activities/

30 Best Mocktail Recipes - Non-Alcoholic Mixed Drinks Ideas https://www.delish.com/entertaining/g3289/mocktail-recipes/

Alcohol and Dopamine https://www.drugrehab.com/addiction/alcohol/alcoholism/alcohol-and-dopamine/

Dry January® Community Group https://www.facebook.com/groups/DryJanuaryCommunity/

Essential Cocktail Preparation Tools for Aspiring Mixologists https://www.curacaoliqueur.com/articles/essential-tools-aspiring-mixologists

Giving Up Alcohol for a Month: 8 Things to Expect https://www.aarp.org/health/healthy-living/info-2024/stop-drinking-for-a-month-benefits.html

How Can I Be an Inspiration in Recovery? | The Guest House https://www.theguesthouseocala.com/how-can-i-be-an-inspiration-in-recovery/

How Much Could You Save By Giving Up Alcohol? https://www.newsweek.com/how-much-money-you-save-giving-alcohol-1848804

How Much Money Will I Save If I Quit Drinking? - Ria Health https://riahealth.com/blog/how-much-money-will-i-save-quit-drinking/#:~:text=The%20Cost%20of%20Drinking,-Photo%20by%20Towfiqu&text=1%20to%203%20drinks%20per,$1,820%20to%20$3,650%20per%20year

How Quitting Alcohol Changes Your Appearance https://oceanrecoverycentre.com/2024/03/how-quitting-alcohol-changes-your-appearance/#:~:text=Skin%20Improvement,common%20sign%20of%20alcohol%20addiction

How To Cope With Social Anxiety Without Alcohol https://riahealth.com/blog/social-anxiety-alcohol/

How to Set and Use SMART Goals https://www.verywellmind.com/smart-goals-for-lifestyle-change-2224097

How to write SMART goals (with examples) https://www.atlassian.com/blog/produc

tivity/how-to-write-smart-goals#:~:text=The%20SMART%20in%20SMART%20goals,within%20a%20certain%20time%20frame

Medical benefits of Dry January and cutting back on alcohol https://www.tebra.com/theintake/medical-deep-dives/tips-and-trends/cheers-to-health-medical-benefits-of-dry-january-and-cutting-back-on-alcohol

Mindfulness Techniques for Addiction Recovery https://lilacrecoverycenter.com/blog/mindfulness-techniques/

Non-Alcoholic Cocktails - The Mindful Mocktail https://mindfulmocktail.com/

Sober-Curious: Benefits of an Alcohol-Free Lifestyle https://www.dulyhealthandcare.com/health-topic/sober-curious-benefits-of-an-alcohol-free-lifestyle#:~:text=Excessive%20alcohol%20consumption%2C%20especially%20over,healthy%20and%20your%20memory%20sharp.

The 10 Best Nonalcoholic Spirits of 2024 https://www.liquor.com/best-non-alcoholic-spirits-5190976

The benefits of "Dry January" last longer than a month, ... https://www.washingtonpost.com/wellness/2022/12/27/dry-january-health-benefits/

The Best Alcohol-Free Events: 30 Tips and Ideas https://www.socialtables.com/blog/event-planning/dry-ideas-alcohol-free-events/

The Craving Cycle: A CBT Concept for Managing Addiction https://yourmindmatters.net.au/the-craving-cycle-a-cbt-concept-for-managing-addiction/

The Dry January® story https://alcoholchange.org.uk/help-and-support/managing-your-drinking/dry-january/about-dry-january/the-dry-january-story

The Mocktail Has Been Here All Along - Punch Drink https://punchdrink.com/articles/mocktail-has-been-here-all-along-historic-non-alcoholic-cocktails/

The Positive Effects of Sobriety on Your Health https://www.aspenhospital.org/healthy-journey/the-positive-effects-of-sobriety-on-your-health/

The Sober Curious Movement Explained https://www.socialrecoverycenter.com/blog/sober-curious-movement#:~:text=The%20%22sober%20curious%22%20movement%20traces,in%20reassessing%20their%20drinking%20habits

The Top Ways Sobriety Improves your Overall Mental Clarity https://www.amyandersontherapy.com/blog/7-ways-sobriety-improves-your-mental-clarity

Tips for Talking With Family About Recovery https://www.providencetreatment.com/addiction-blog/tips-talking-family-recovery/

Tools and Apps to Track Money Saved by Drinking Less https://www.joinreframeapp.com/blog-post/tools-and-apps-to-track-money-saved-by-drinking-less

Try Dry®: the app for Dry January® and beyond https://alcoholchange.org.uk/help-and-support/managing-your-drinking/dry-january/get-involved/the-dry-january-app

ABOUT THE PUBLISHER

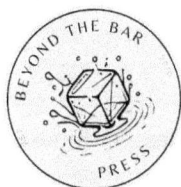

With over two decades of experience in the alcohol beverage industry, Beyond the Bar Press has established itself as a trusted and innovative publisher dedicated to transforming how we perceive and enjoy beverages. Founded by industry veterans who recognized the evolving landscape of social drinking and the growing movement towards mindful consumption, Beyond the Bar Press has consistently delivered insightful, engaging, and practical resources for enthusiasts and those seeking a healthier, more intentional relationship with alcohol.

Beyond the Bar Press was born out of a deep understanding of the multifaceted impacts of alcohol on individuals and communities. Our founders, having worked in various facets of the beverage industry, gained firsthand insight into the cultural, social, and health-related aspects of alcohol consumption. This extensive background provided a unique perspective that blends industry expertise with a compassionate approach to personal well-being, ensuring our audience feels understood and cared for.

As the "sober curious" movement continues to gain momentum, Beyond the Bar Press saw an opportunity to support and empower individuals exploring a life with less or no alcohol. Recognizing the need for quality resources that offer both inspiration and practical guidance, the publisher shifted its focus to creating content that caters to this growing audience. Their mission is to provide readers with the knowledge and tools to make informed choices about their drinking habits, while still enjoying the social and creative aspects of beverage preparation and consumption.

Beyond the Bar Press also strongly emphasizes innovation and creativity. Understanding that one of the joys of social drinking is experimenting with flavors and presentation, their publications often feature unique recipes and tips for elevating non-alcoholic beverages to new heights. By highlighting familiar favorite flavors alongside unconventional ingredients, they encourage readers to explore and expand their palates without the need for alcohol. This approach makes the transition to mindful drinking enjoyable and enhances the overall drinking experience.

Looking ahead, Beyond the Bar Press continues to innovate and expand its offerings, staying attuned to the latest trends and developments in the beverage industry and the sober curious movement. Our unwavering dedication to helping others navigate the complexities of alcohol consumption and embrace a more intentional lifestyle ensures our audience feels informed and up-to-date.

www.ingramcontent.com/pod-product-compliance
Lightning Source LLC
Chambersburg PA
CBHW070125030426
42335CB00016B/2275